Let's Have Healthy Children

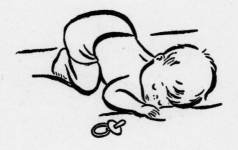

BY ADELLE DAVIS, A.B., M.S.

CONSULTING NUTRITIONIST

HARCOURT, BRACE AND COMPANY: NEW YORK

PRINTED IN THE UNITED STATES OF AMERICA

Dedicated

to

Our Two Chosen Children

GEORDIE AND BARBIE

Without Whose Cooperation

This Book Would Never Have Been Written

PREFACE

IN NUTRITION, the gap between knowing and doing is distressingly wide; it allows imperfect growth and development and results in the needless production of almost every degree of ill health. The author hopes that this book may help to narrow the gap.

To the many persons who have aided in the preparation of the manuscript or who have offered valuable criticisms, the author wishes to express her thanks: Mrs. Bernice Hicks, Dr. Arthur C. Hicks, Mrs. Leah D. Widtsoe, Mrs. Dolly Connelly, Mrs. Barbara Hall, Mrs. Horace J. Smith, Mrs. Robert Ingram, Mrs. Helen J. Graham, Mrs. Frank Vukmanic, Mrs. Beatrice Woodbridge, and Miss Olive Burchfiel. Outstandingly helpful have been the following physicians who have given generously of their time and have offered excellent criticisms of the entire manuscript or the parts pertaining to their specialty: Dr. Harold L. Snow, Dr. Vincent J. Rounds, Dr. Lowell R. Hill, Dr. Joseph C. Risser, and Dr. Robert Null.

The author also gratefully acknowledges her indebtedness to Marilyn and Egon Reich for the drawings used throughout the book.

ADELLE DAVIS LEISEY

TABLE OF CONTENTS

ix

Let's Have Healthy Children

CHAPTER 1

IS A GOOD DIET DURING
PREGNANCY WORTH WHILE?

YOU'RE going to have a baby. What joys are in store for you! A thousand thrills will be yours which perhaps no one else can share: yours is the thrill of holding your baby for the first time; of stroking his head; of feeling the push of his little button nose into your neck; and of experiencing the viselike grasp of his tiny hands around your fingers. To others he may seem unattractive and even to you momentarily, but he becomes more beautiful each minute.

You will watch him purse his lips, mouth open in birdlike fashion, as he gropes for his first meal. You will enjoy the hundreds of vague noises he makes: the squeaky sounds of satisfaction after he has been fed, almost like the creaking of a new leather saddle; the tiny rusty-hinge noises; the little piglike grunts; and the cooings of contentment. The first beginnings of a smile will probably be yours to enjoy alone. And if you are healthy and truly feminine, holding your baby to your breast and letting him nurse his fill will probably be the ultimate satisfaction of your motherhood.

There are thrills of motherhood which you will have aside from your baby. You will enjoy your own confidence, knowing that you are going to be a good mother to this child. You will enjoy the vigor of your own strong body, driving you to fulfill the baby's needs. You will experience the fun of "playing dolls" all over again. You will enjoy rocking your baby, singing him lullabies, and talking to him in language he probably understands far more than we realize. You will thank God that what

3

was once called spoiling a baby is now known to give him a feeling of security which can last throughout his lifetime.

If your nutrition has been adequate throughout pregnancy and your general health is good, what can we expect of this new baby of yours? We can, of course, expect him to be perfectly formed and free from physical defects. We can expect him to lift his head momentarily as if looking around to see what he thinks of this world he has entered. We can expect his eyes to open wide and be well focused and co-ordinated, although unseeing. You need not be surprised if his tiny legs, held in the right position, will brace themselves, even giving a miniature jump at times. If you put the baby on his face in crib or bassinet, he may even "crawl" to the head of his bed. The skin on his scalp will be beautifully clean and attractive. His sucking reflexes will be amazingly strong, and he will have no trouble in taking the nipple. If his needs are fulfilled, as they should be, you will probably be surprised how seldom he cries.

Such is the picture of a well-nourished mother who has brought into the world a well-nourished baby. Unfortunately the picture is often different indeed. The exhausted and undernourished mother can almost hate this ugly thing which has caused her such pain. She may be irritated by his crying and suffer pain from his nursing, her nipples perhaps cracked and bleeding. Her confidence is crowded out by fears and worries. She may be afraid to pick up her baby or to wash his scalp thoroughly. Every spitting up of milk or change of texture in the stools may indicate to her possible illness and make her fly in fear to phone her doctor. Tension replaces relaxation, and she probably looks forward to night feeding with dread.

Her infant, born undernourished, cannot compare with the healthy one. His head wobbles. His eyes are not co-ordinated or well focused. His eyelids may rarely open at first. His head may be covered with unsightly "scalp cap." He is not able to brace his feet, to "crawl" in the crib, or to lift his head easily. His sucking reflexes may be so weak that he cannot nurse strongly enough to stimulate normal milk flow. In fact, he may even refuse to take the breast. He probably cries irritably much of the time. He may not only be in poor general physical condition but be born with one or more congenital defects.

It now appears that every woman, by her choice of foods during pregnancy, largely determines the type of baby she will produce. Although hundreds of studies, both with pregnant women and with experimental animals, help to justify such a statement, particularly outstanding is the research of two groups. One study was made by a group of doctors from the School of Public Health at Harvard University,[1] working at the prenatal clinics of the Boston Lying-in Hospital; and the other by doctors from the Departments of Obstetrics and Pediatrics of the University of Toronto Medical School.[2] In each case, detailed information was gathered concerning the food eaten by the women when they first reported at the prenatal clinics, usually during their fourth month of pregnancy, and continuously afterward until their babies were born.

In the Harvard study, 216 women were classed into five groups according to their diets: excellent, good, fair, poor, and very poor. The report does not give details of the food eaten but only the analysis of the diet the physicians considered excellent (p. 22).

The Toronto doctors divided their expectant mothers, 400 in all, into three groups according to the diets they had followed: poor diets, good diets, and poor diets supplemented to good. In this study, money was available to help some of the women who could not afford nutritious food. Of the expectant mothers coming to the clinic alternate patients whose diets were poor were put into a group which would receive supplements. An egg, an orange, and 1 quart of milk were delivered daily to each patient of the latter group; 1 pound of cheese, a few cans of tomatoes,

---

[1] B. S. Burke, V. A. Beal, S. A. Kirkwood, and H. C. Stuart, "Nutritional Studies During Pregnancy," *American Journal of Obstetrics and Gynecology,* 46 (1943), 38.

[2] J. H. Ebbs, F. F. Tisdall, and W. A. Scott, "The Influence of Prenatal Diet on the Mother and Child," *Journal of Nutrition,* 22 (1941), 515.

and a package of wheat germ were delivered each week. The women were supplied with capsules containing 2,000 units of vitamin D to be taken daily. A social worker called at the homes to see that other members of the family were not eating the food provided. The women were asked to have at least half of their breads and cereal of whole grains, and to use only iodized salt.

Babies are healthier when the mothers' diets have been good. In both the Toronto and Harvard studies, the infants were examined by pediatricians who were unaware of the quality of the food eaten by the mothers. When the prenatal diets were correlated with the condition of the infants, the Harvard group found that 87 per cent of the mothers whose diets had been adequate gave birth to infants in good or excellent condition. Another 10 per cent of the babies had only minor counts against them such as mild inflammation of the eyes or small umbilical hernias. Only one infant of the entire group was defective; he had a congenital heart condition.

In contrast, when the mothers' diets had been particularly inadequate, 95 per cent of the infants were found to be in poor or extremely poor physical condition. The group in extremely poor condition included infants who were stillborn; infants who died a few hours or days after birth (one died of bronchitis and another of bronchopneumonia when 3 days old); feeble-minded and mentally retarded babies; and infants with cleft palates, congenital heart defects, and congenital cataract. (See page 19.) The group in poor condition included babies with such abnormalities as tumors, clubbed feet, crossed eyes and other eye abnormalities, and several infants suffering from thrush and severe skin infections. Many of these infants were born prematurely. Of all the infants of the women whose diets had been poor, only one was judged to be in excellent health and another in good condition.

The findings of the Toronto doctors were similar. When the mothers' diet was poor, more than 3 per cent of the babies were born dead, whereas no stillbirths occurred among women whose diets had been good. Four times as many babies were born prematurely to women whose diets had been poor as to the women whose diets were adequate.

Labor is easier when the prenatal diet has been good. The Toronto doctors found that women whose diets had been poor had difficult labor, whereas fewer women who had eaten more adequately had difficulty (24 per cent compared with 3 per cent). Yet the women on the poorer diet gave birth to twice as many premature infants, who were naturally smaller than full-term babies. More of the poorly fed women suffered hemorrhages during labor, and three times as many contracted infections of the uterus. Twice as many suffered from breast infections, and three times as many had breast abscesses.

The Harvard group also found that, in spite of the fact that the babies were much smaller, labor was more difficult and the complications far more severe when women had eaten a poor diet during their pregnancy. The actual hours of labor for women having their first babies was the same in both groups, but for women who had had one or more children, the hours of labor were found to have decreased almost to half when the diets had been good. The women having more adequate diets suffered fewer hemorrhages and lacerations, and their uterine contractions were stronger. The poorly fed women convalesced more slowly, and three times as many suffered from such major complications as severe hemorrhages; infections of the uterus and urinary tract; phlebitis; high blood pressure; and inflammations, infections, and abscesses of the breast as did the better-fed women.

Pregnancy is more normal when the diet is good. The Toronto group found that almost six times as many women on an inadequate diet had poor health during pregnancy compared with that of women staying on a good diet. Almost twice as many of the poor-diet group suffered from severe anemia, eight times as many were threatened with miscarriage, and twice as many suffered from toxemia. None of the group having the better food had miscarriages, whereas 6 per cent of the inadequate-diet group miscarried.

The Harvard study revealed that when the women stayed on a good diet, about a third (32 per cent) suffered complications during pregnancy; their principal complications were nausea and staining, or threatened miscarriage. Of the women on poor diets, 58 per cent suffered complications, which were often severe. Almost half of these women suffered from toxemia (p. 48), whereas none of those on good diets developed toxemia.

An expectant mother can appear to be healthy; yet her baby may be abnormal. A striking fact was brought out by the Harvard study: many of the inadequately fed women appeared to be in good health during their pregnancy but gave birth to infants who were in extremely poor physical condition. In fact, 42 per cent of these women progressed satisfactorily during pregnancy; yet only 5 per cent of all the babies in this group were in good condition. Until recently there has been a general belief that a pregnant woman's health was sacrificed for her infant and that if the mother was progressing satisfactorily, her baby would be healthy. The Harvard doctors point out: "It may be entirely possible that a woman may run an apparently satisfactory clinical course, but if she is consuming an inadequate diet, the fetus will suffer."

Mothers whose diets are good during pregnancy have more chance to nurse their babies. The Toronto group [3] found that when a mother's diet had been good during pregnancy, she not only secreted more milk but could nurse her baby much longer than could a woman whose diet had been inadequate. By the time the babies were 6 weeks old, three times as many women from the poor-diet group were bottle feeding their infants. When supplementary foods were no longer delivered to the homes, the diets of the mothers became so inadequate that only a few of them could continue nursing their babies.

[3] J. H. Ebbs and H. Kelly, "The Relation of the Maternal Diet During Pregnancy to Breast Feeding," *Archives of the Diseases of Childhood*, **16** (1942), 212.

Although the Harvard group does not report the effect of the diets upon breast feedings, much other research indicates that a mother's ability to nurse her infant is determined largely by her diet before the baby is born.

When the prenatal diets had been good, the babies stayed healthier. The Toronto group found that by the time the babies were 6 months old, five times as many whose mothers had been on an inadequate prenatal diet had suffered from frequent colds as did infants whose mothers' diets had been good before their birth. Three times as many infants from the poor-diet group had suffered from bronchitis, four times as many had had pneumonia, almost three times as many were anemic, and six times as many were dystrophic (had failed to grow normally). None of the infants whose mothers had stayed on the good diet had rickets, whereas a number of the poor-diet infants not only had severe rickets but also had convulsions (tetany) caused by poor absorption of calcium. Three of the infants whose mothers' diets had been faulty died before they were 6 months old, whereas there were no deaths in the other group.

The Harvard group also found that there were more infections among the babies whose mothers' diets had been poor. The increased incidence of infections occurred particularly during the second half of the first year of life.

Advantages omitted by research. An extremely important factor which was omitted by these studies is the effect of diet upon the mother's emotions and upon her home life. A young mother whose prenatal diet had been excellent recently phoned me soon after her delivery.

"I feel wonderful," she exclaimed. "My delivery was a breeze, but it kills me to have to stay in the hospital for 4 more days. I'm dying to get home to Frank and to take care of my baby."

I saw a great deal of this happy mother, her fine young husband, and their beautiful infant. Never once did I hear of worries or complaints of fatigue, nor did I see signs of tension or irritability to mar the graciousness of their home.

In contrast was another young mother whose income was more

than adequate but whose diet was atrocious. She was ill during much of her pregnancy and far from well afterward. She worried constantly, was depressed and easily angered, and frequently sobbed without knowing why. Her infant had colic for weeks, and although kept under barbiturates, cried piteously much of the time. The young husband, worried sick and exhausted from lack of sleep, dropped in to see me and blew his top. Having that baby was a frightful mistake. He hated the squalling thing. It had ruined Dorothy's health. Their married life had gone to pieces. She cared nothing for him now, only for the baby.

Tension and irritability, depression and uncontrollable weeping have all been produced in persons who have volunteered to stay on inadequate diets, particularly diets deficient in almost any one of the many B vitamins. Lack of graciousness in the home can be the result of an inadequate diet just as much as can an infant born in poor physical condition.

An adequate prenatal diet is worth while. That an adequate prenatal diet is worth while can no longer be doubted. Many fine obstetricians are fully aware of its value and make every effort to keep their patients on adequate diets. Unfortunately other obstetricians have little interest in nutrition and believe that a "well-balanced diet"—whatever that means—supplies everything the expectant mother needs. Such doctors sometimes recommend inadequate diets which may actually produce illnesses in the mother and abnormalities in her infant.

There are also thousands of conscientious women who are eager to do everything in their power to insure that the child they carry will be healthy and intelligent. There are other women who eat as they please regardless of the effect upon themselves or their infants, although they may be able to afford the best food available. If they are ill during their pregnancies or their infants are defective in one way or another, such, they believe, are the accidents of nature.

The Harvard group, in summarizing the report, made this statement: "There can be no doubt from these findings that, if the mother's diet during pregnancy is poor to very poor, she will in all probability have a poor infant from the standpoint of physical condition. If the mother has a good or excellent diet, she will probably have an infant in good or excellent condition."

You, as an intelligent expectant mother, can produce the type of infant which will make you proud and happy that your diet was adequate during your pregnancy.

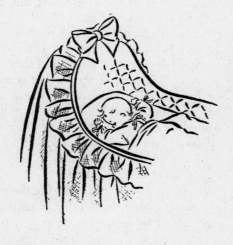

CHAPTER 2

START BEFORE CONCEPTION
TO PREPARE FOR YOUR BABY

D URING the past years many fine young women have come
to consult me, often with their husbands, and have told me
that they are ready to start rearing their families but wish to be
in as nearly perfect health as possible before they become pregnant. Frequently they have talked about a sister or friend who
has been particularly ill during pregnancy, and they wish to avoid
a similar experience. To follow an adequate diet is not difficult for
these girls. They have a goal which thrills them and is worth
working for. They will not be fighting nausea, as perhaps they
might if they waited to improve their diets after they became
pregnant. Regardless of how unpleasant a food may taste, if that
food supplies nutrients which will eventually help their babies,
they have been good sports about eating it.

I have seen these young women again during their pregnancies.
Most of them have never experienced a day of nausea. They have
rarely had to worry about threatened miscarriage. Instead of the
dozens of complaints one usually hears from a group of expectant
mothers, these girls almost invariably make the remark, "I've
never felt better in my life!" Not one of them has given birth to
a premature, stillborn, or malformed child.

In due time they come in with their babies, and what beautiful
babies they are! It is difficult to say who is more proud of them,
their parents or I. Such experiences are satisfying indeed.

Improve your diet before conception. Thousands of experiments with animals show that the health of the parents prior to
conception is an important factor in determining the strength and

well-being of the young. Studies indicate that if your diet is consistently adequate both before your child is conceived and afterward, the chances are not only that you will produce a superior infant but that you will avoid the illnesses so common during pregnancy.

Usually a woman eats whatever food she happens to enjoy. Probably she suffers a number of mild nutritional deficiencies; perhaps her blood pressure or blood count is a bit low; she may have an occasional bout with constipation or headaches now and again; she has some tooth decay, her gums may bleed a little, and she bruises easily; she perhaps suffers from a few colds or a mild sinus infection or has a touch of hay fever in season. She considers herself healthy, however, because of her low standards.

In this condition she conceives and is perhaps aware of conception only after nausea sets in. Even though the nausea is mild, it is almost impossible for her to eat an adequate diet during this period. Her deficiencies become more severe, while her nutritional requirements greatly increase. The nausea perhaps lasts for 3 months and may develop into pernicious vomiting. Even if she follows an excellent diet during the remainder of her pregnancy, it is almost impossible for her to obtain sufficient nutrients to overcome the deficiencies in herself, to meet her current needs, and to supply all the requirements of her growing infant. Her chances of producing a really superior baby were sacrificed *before* she conceived.

Several babies in close succession. The other day I saw a mother with a boy 3 years old, a girl 11 months younger, and a baby of a few months. The boy was a beautiful child, the girl a pathetic little thing, and the baby, who had been ill since birth, was a sad picture indeed. The mother told me, with apparent surprise, that the oldest child had been so easy to care for, the second one had been considerable trouble, and the third had caused them constant worry and anxiety. You can find hundreds of similar examples if you look for them.

When a mother is fairly healthy, and her diet, although unplanned, happens to be more or less adequate, her first baby is usually a fine, normal infant. He has, however, probably robbed her body of any calcium, phosphorus, and iron which may have been stored. Unless her diet has been excellent, the increased requirements of pregnancy have left her with multiple subtle deficiencies. In this condition, she again conceives. She is so busy taking care of her first baby that she has little time to prepare food for herself. Chances are the budget is more limited, and she "economizes" by buying less expensive foods. Furthermore, her confidence has soared because she has produced a healthy infant without special attention to diet, and she feels she can do it again. Her deficiencies become more severe and more difficult to overcome; the second baby is less healthy than the first. Thus each successive child is probably born more and more undernourished. Yet the mother rarely recognizes that she, herself, has needlessly robbed her younger children of their birthright, that of a healthy body.

If you wish to have your children in close succession, keep your diet unusually adequate not only during but between pregnancies. With each successive child, adhere to a nutritious diet still more rigidly. Know that your own requirements are increased not only by the demands of pregnancy but also by your greater physical activity necessary in caring for your babies.

Trouble during a previous pregnancy. If during a previous pregnancy you have had trouble which may have been caused by dietary deficiencies, it becomes extremely important to stay on a completely adequate diet for 3 months or longer before you conceive again. Perhaps you experienced unusually severe nausea; perhaps threatened miscarriage made it necessary for you to remain in bed for weeks; perhaps you developed toxemia; or perhaps your baby was born prematurely and had to be kept in an incubator when you were longing to care for him yourself, even though he was a weak, whimpering infant. If dietary deficiencies have caused these abnormalities and are not corrected, the chances are that they will become even more severe during another pregnancy. Instead of nausea you may experience pernicious vomiting; instead of threatened miscarriage you may have an actual miscarriage; instead of toxemia you may develop eclampsia; instead of a premature birth your next child may be stillborn. The outlook is not a happy one.

On the other hand, if your diet is more than adequate prior to conception and during pregnancy, these abnormalities may not occur. I can recall several women who had suffered pernicious vomiting with previous pregnancies; yet by improving their diets before the next conception, they did not experience a day of nausea. Two women whom I remember had four and five miscarriages, respectively, yet they gave birth to beautiful children after their preconception and pregnancy diets were improved. Anyone working in nutrition can tell you of women who went into eclampsia with one pregnancy; then by improving their diets they experienced no difficulty with a following pregnancy. I recently saw a woman who had suffered severe nausea during two pregnancies and each time had developed toxemia and given birth to premature infants. After the birth of her second baby, she became interested in nutrition and kept herself on an unusually adequate diet. A third pregnancy resulted in fine twin girls who were born 2 weeks overdue, a rare occurrence indeed. Twins are usually born prematurely because the nutritional demands on the mother are so great that no ordinary diet can meet the requirements.

Difficulty in conceiving. Malnutrition on the part of either the husband or wife may prevent conception. Experiments have shown that vitamin-A deficiency can markedly lower fertility. It has been proved that the B vitamins and adequate proteins are essential to the normal production of both ovum and sperm; that without these nutrients fewer sperm and ova are produced; and that the sperm lack motility. A mild deficiency of vitamin E may cause fewer sperm to be produced, and a severe deficiency causes sterility in the male.

If you have difficulty in conceiving, go with your husband to a good gynecologist. In addition to following his advice, it is important that both you and your husband stay on the best diet you can. Since the diet for pregnancy (p. 35) is planned to be adequate in all known nutrients, it can serve as a guide for you to follow.

If your sterility should remain cruelly permanent, by all means adopt a baby. An Italian woman said to me recently, "When you havva no babies, you havva nothing." How right she is!

Prevent nausea now. Although the causes are not completely understood, nausea appears to result principally from an undersupply of protein and of the B vitamins. Eat the foods rich in these nutrients (pp. 24, 29) until they come out of your ears. Since the B vitamins are not stored in the body but must be obtained daily, be even more conscientious about eating these foods after you become pregnant. If your diet is adequate, your chances of preventing nausea are excellent.

Try to prevent miscarriage before conception. In all probability every nutrient plays some role in helping to carry through a normal pregnancy. It has long been known that a lack of vitamin E causes experimental animals to miscarry soon after conception. The value of vitamin E in preventing miscarriage in humans, however, is still bitterly disputed. Despite the disagreement, evidence points to the fact that an adequate intake of this vitamin should be obtained. Dr. Bacharach [1] cites a study of 81 women who had had a total of 227 previous miscarriages. They were given 6 milligrams of vitamin E daily in the form of wheat-germ oil for 3 to 32 weeks. With this treatment, the next 81 pregnancies resulted in 62 living infants. In another study, after treatment with vitamin E, 72 women who had experienced recurrent miscarriages, some as many as 4 and 5, gave birth to 55 healthy infants. Dr. Vogt-Möller, an obstetrician who has spent two decades in research on the value of vitamin E, wrote as early as 1939: "The records of treated cases of habitual abortion now amount to some hundreds with a mean value of 75 to 80 per cent favorable results." [2]

---

[1] A. L. Bacharach, "Vitamin E and Habitual Abortion," *British Medical Journal*, 1 (1940), 890.

[2] *Vitamin E. A Symposium.* Society of Chemical Industry, London, 1939.

Dr. Young,[3] professor of obstetrics at the University of London Medical School, points out that to be of value vitamin E should be generously supplied before the placenta is formed. Since the placenta starts to grow almost immediately after conception, it is wise to see that your diet is rich in vitamin E before conception. The richest sources of vitamin E are wheat germ and wheat-germ oil. Concentrates of vitamin E, prepared by distilling salad oils, are now available which are hundreds of times more potent than wheat germ. The amount of the vitamin which may prevent miscarriage is not known. The quantities used for treatment have varied from 6 to as much as 270 milligrams daily. Wheat germ, however, should be eaten for its other nutrients as well as for the vitamin E it supplies.

Can malformations be prevented? Probably all expectant mothers worry at some time for fear their babies will be malformed. Evidence is accumulating which indicates that it may be possible to prevent malformations rather than merely worry about them.

The relationship between the maternal diet and malformations in the young of animals was first shown by research conducted at the Texas Agricultural Experimental Station.[4] Vitamin-A deficiencies were produced in sows before they were bred. The little pigs were born without eyeballs, and a large proportion had hare-lips, cleft palates, and abnormally formed ears. In one case, a sow was so weak before breeding that some vitamin A had to be given. The pigs had eyeballs but were blind.

Since that time, a wide variety of experimental animals put on diets deficient in vitamin A have produced young showing almost every type of malformation: blindness; deafness; clubbed feet; cleft palates; harelips; and anomalies (malformations) of the heart, kidneys, lungs, diaphragm, and testicles. Dr. Warkany [5]

[3] J. Young, "The Habitual Abortion and Stillbirth Syndrome and Late Pregnancy Toxemia," *Brit. Med. J.*, 1 (1937), 953.

[4] F. Hale, "The Relation of Vitamin A to Anophthalmos in Pigs," *American Journal of Ophthalmology*, 18 (1935), 1087.

[5] J. Warkany and C. B. Roth, "Congenital Malformations Induced in Rats by Maternal Vitamin-A Deficiency," *J. Nutrition*, 35 (1948), 1.

and his associates have produced malformations of almost every type in rats by putting the mothers, prior to mating, on diets lacking either vitamin A or vitamin B_2. All of the animals have defective eyes when vitamin A is undersupplied, and 75 per cent have heart lesions [6] and abnormalities of the kidneys. The eyes of the young are also particularly affected when the maternal diet has lacked vitamin B_2, although only about 50 per cent of these animals develop gross abnormalities. If the diet is made rich in the missing nutrient during the first few days after conception, the malformations can sometimes be prevented.

Whether malformations are produced in human infants by inadequate maternal diets is not known. Furthermore, it is almost impossible to study the preconception diets of mothers of malformed children; too much time has elapsed before the malformations become apparent. Dr. Laudtman,[7] working at the University College Hospital in London, however, searched the prenatal histories of mothers whose children had been born blind or deaf or had suffered such malformations as clubbed feet, congenital heart disease, anomalies of the kidneys or diaphragm, and defective brains such as anencephaly (monster without a brain). He found that more than one-fifth of the mothers at the very beginning of pregnancy had suffered acute infections such as flu, severe colds, bronchitis, pneumonia, or kidney infections. That an inadequate diet can lower resistance and be a causative factor in the susceptibility to such infections is established.

Doctors from the University of Pennsylvania Medical School [8] undertook a study of the prenatal diets of mothers who had given birth to 545 children so malformed that 90 per cent were born dead or died within a year after birth. Medical students went

[6] J. Warkany and J. A. Wilson, "Cardiac Anomalies in the Offspring of Vitamin-A-Deficient Rats," *American Journal of Anatomy*, 85 (1928), 113, 357.

[7] B. Laudtman, "On the Relationship between Maternal Conditions During Pregnancy and Congenital Malformations," *Arch. Dis. Childhood*, 23 (1948), 237.

[8] D. P. Murphy and A. Deplant, "Food Habits of Mothers of Congenitally Malformed Children," *Am. J. Obst. Gynec.*, 37 (1939), 460.

into the homes and interviewed each mother, obtaining as much detailed information about her food habits as was possible. The diets of these women were found to have been deficient in practically every nutrient. Almost half of them had drunk no milk at all, and only 1 per cent had taken as much as a quart daily. More than 80 per cent of them ate only white bread. So few fresh fruits and vegetables had been used that the diets were considered to have been markedly deficient in iron and in vitamins A, B_2, and C. Although the information collected applied to diets during pregnancy, there is no reason to believe that their nutrition was better before conception.

An inadequate maternal diet, however, is certainly not the only cause of malformed infants. It has long been known that if a woman suffers from German measles at any time during the first 3 months of pregnancy or if she has syphilis, she may give birth to a malformed child. Evidence suggests, however, that certain malformations might be prevented if a woman's diet is adequate both before conception and during pregnancy.

See your physician before you become pregnant. Whenever possible, go to your physician for a general physical examination before you become pregnant. Ask him what your blood count and blood pressure are, and if they deviate from normal, take steps to correct them (pp. 50, 52). At least try to correct any deviations from health which he may discover. If you have not done so already, this is a good time to make a study of nutrition. Read a number of books on the subject and learn to recognize symptoms of deficiencies and measures for correcting them.

No book on nutrition can meet the needs of every person. The more you learn about nutrition, however, the more you will be able to select foods rich in the nutrients which you, as an individual, may lack or need in larger than usual quantities. The prenatal diet (p. 35), planned to supply adequate amounts of all known nutrients, can serve as a guide.

The best diet, however, cannot overcome the harm done by years of living on cokes, coffee, cigarettes, and products made from white flour and refined sugar. The longer your diet has been inadequate and the more inadequate it has been, the longer you should stay on an excellent diet before conceiving.

Any woman who will make the effort will find that adherence to an excellent preconception diet pays rich dividends.

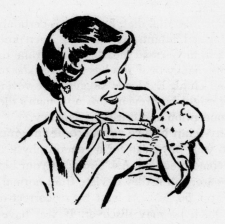

CHAPTER 3

YOUR DIET DURING PREGNANCY

A T NO time during life are your nutritional requirements so high as when you are pregnant or are nursing your baby. If you are to stay well and your infant is to be physically superior, your nutritional requirements must be met. Nature deals cruelly with any carelessness or failure.

There are only a few general rules to follow in planning any diet: all known nutrients must be supplied; foods should be largely unrefined so that unknown nutrients may be included; any nutrient which has been lacking should be obtained in more than ample amounts until the deficiency is overcome. Even when a diet is completely adequate, nutrients may be destroyed in the body, may not be efficiently absorbed into the blood, or may be lost through urine or feces. Malnutrition is the result of deficiencies of essential nutrients in the tissue cells rather than in the diet.

Minimum versus optimum requirements. Standards have been set up giving recommended daily allowances of the better known nutrients. Three such standards are given on page 22. In planning dietary recommendations, however, the ability of persons to pay for foods supplying the nutrients must be considered. The Food and Nutrition Board of the National Research Council, in planning dietary allowances for everyone in the United States, was forced to consider the many families whose total annual income was $300 or less. Dr. Dieckmann,[1] chief of staff at the Chicago Lying-in Hospital, points out that he wants expectant

[1] W. J. Dieckmann, "Diet from the Viewpoint of the Obstetrician," *Nutrition Reviews,* **6** (1948), 129.

RECOMMENDED DIETARY ALLOWANCES

	Calories	Protein grams	Calcium grams	Iron mg.
National Research Council				
Pregnancy	2,500	85	1.5	15
Lactation	3,000	100	2.0	15
Boston Lying-in Hospital *				
Pregnancy	2,600-2,800	85-100	1.5	20
Chicago Lying-in Hospital				
Pregnancy	⁻1,800	85-125 †	1.4	16
Optimum amounts suggested by author				
Pregnancy	2,200	100-125	2-3	20
Lactation	2,500	125-150	3	20

mg. = milligrams.   * See ref. 1, p. 5.   † Explained in text.

mothers to obtain 125 grams of protein daily although they can rarely afford as much as 85 grams. Such standards, therefore, meet minimum rather than ideal requirements.

You do not apply minimum standards in buying a car, a house, or even an item costing a few pennies. Why should you use minimum standards in planning anything as valuable as health, particularly when you are creating a new life? Dr. Sherman, formerly professor of food chemistry at Columbia University, proved years ago that by giving experimental animals a minimum amount of vitamin A, all appearances of health could be maintained. If that amount was doubled, tripled, or quadrupled, however, the animals showed greater evidences of health with each increase. Dr. Sherman recommends that every person get at least 10,000 units daily of vitamin A and preferably 20,000 units. He would be the first to grant that the need for this vitamin is still further increased by pregnancy. Similarly Dr. Szent Györgyi, who was awarded the Nobel prize for his research in vitamin C, pointed out that experimental animals could be kept apparently healthy when a few milligrams of vitamin C were given them daily. If they were to

DURING PREGNANCY AND LACTATION

Vitamin A units	Vitamin B₁ mg.	Vitamin B₂ mg.	Niacin mg.	Vitamin C mg.	Vitamin D units
6,000	1.8	2.5	18	100	400
8,000	2.0	3.0	20	150	400
8,000	2.0	2.5	18	100	400-800
20,337	1.6	2.9	18	139	400-800
25,000	4-5	6	50	300	2,000-3,000
50,000	5	7	60	300	2,000-3,000

be unharmed by bacterial toxins, however, twenty times that amount of vitamin C was required.

Because of such experimental evidence I recommend daily allowances considerably higher than those of other standards. The diets I have recommended to expectant mothers for years have met these standards; the women who have followed such diets carefully have kept in excellent health, and their infants, in my opinion, are far superior to those whose mothers have eaten foods supplying fewer nutrients.

Unfortunately, space cannot be given to tell why each nutrient is needed or how each is used to maintain health. Such information can be found in *Vitality Through Planned Nutrition* [2] and a number of other popular books on the subject.

Meeting your protein requirement. Your first concern must be to obtain adequate protein. The entire structure of your growing baby's body will be made of the proteins you eat. At the same time you will need protein to keep your own muscles, vital organs,

[2] Adelle Davis, *Vitality Through Planned Nutrition* (2d ed.; New York: The Macmillan Company, 1949).

and other body tissues in constant repair and to produce hormones, enzymes, antibodies, and blood cells for yourself. You must also obtain enough protein to form new tissue in your uterus and breasts.

The proteins you eat will be broken down during digestion into 22 different amino acids. These amino acids will be used to repair body structures and to build new tissues. Ten of the amino acids cannot be made in the body; it is as necessary to obtain them from foods as it is to obtain the vitamins. In fact, your health during pregnancy and the very life of your baby may be determined by the adequacy of a single essential amino acid in your diet.

To eat enough protein is so important that you should memorize the quantities in the foods given in the following table. Know these figures so thoroughly that each night before you go to bed,

Food	Amount	Protein grams
Whole milk	1 quart	33
Skim milk	1 quart	34
Powdered skim milk	½ cup, rounded, or 10 tablespoons	35
Egg	1	6
Brewers' yeast	1 heaping tablespoon, or 45 grams	20
Peanut butter	2 tablespoons	9
Prepared cereals (cornflakes, bran flakes, etc.)	1 serving	2-3
Cooked cereal (oatmeal, ground wheat, etc.)	1 serving	5-7
Wheat germ, raw or toasted	½ cup, rounded	24
Cottage cheese	½ cup	20
American or Swiss cheese	1 serving	10-12
Meat, fish, or fowl	1 serving	12-24
Macaroni, noodles, or rice	1 serving	3-4
Navy or lima beans	1 serving	6-8
Soybeans	1 serving	20
Whole-wheat bread	1 slice	3
Bacon	1 slice lean	2

you can in a second mentally calculate the grams of protein you have eaten during the day; if the quantity is inadequate, eat protein-rich foods before retiring. The amounts of protein in still other foods are given in the tables on pages 278 to 293. You will notice that such foods as gelatin and many fresh vegetables contain proteins, but these proteins either lack so many essential amino acids or are so small in amount that they are not worth considering.

I recently checked the diet of a young woman in her seventh month of pregnancy. She believed she was eating a high-protein diet because she had an egg each morning, luncheon meat or a fourth of a cup of cottage cheese at noon, and meat or fish at dinner. She was actually getting about 40 grams of protein daily, or less than half of her minimum requirement. Unless you actually count the grams of protein you eat daily, the chances are that you will obtain far too little of this valuable nutrient and that your baby will be inferior to what he could have been.

Usually a high-protein diet is so expensive that few expectant mothers can afford it. Such a diet can be planned, however, which is economical. One of the least expensive proteins of the highest quality is supplied by powdered skim milk. A pound of this milk costing 14 cents (p. 261) furnishes more than 140 grams of protein which, if obtained from steaks, would cost at least $7.

All expectant mothers should drink at least a quart of milk daily; since weight must be controlled, skim milk is usually preferable. I recommend that about a cup of fresh milk be poured into a bowl, an electric beater, or a liquefier (the easiest method), then a generous ½ cup of powdered skim milk put *on top* of the liquid and beaten until smooth; pour this milk mixture into a bottle or quart jar, and as soon as the foam disintegrates, fill the bottle or jar with the remainder of the quart of fresh milk. By this method, the protein content of the milk has been increased from 34 grams to 69 grams. If the budget is limited, 1¼ cups of powdered skim milk can be beaten with an equal amount of water and poured into a milk bottle or quart jar, which can then be filled with water. When chilled, this reconstructed milk is not unpalatable. Powdered milk can also be added to cooked cereals, gravies, cream soups and sauces, custards, puddings, junkets, and dozens of other foods.[3] It can be purchased directly from many dairies, often from small bakeries, and from health-food stores. If you use it, keep it dry in airtight containers.

Aside from milk, however, eat any proteins you enjoy and can afford. Just make sure you eat enough of them.

Meeting your calcium requirements. Fresh and powdered milk are the only dependable sources of calcium. Even cheese is not a reliable source because the calcium is usually lost in the whey during cheese making. The requirements of calcium are increased by pregnancy, particularly during the last 3 months. Although the amount of calcium needed can be obtained if the diet is carefully chosen, most obstetricians wisely recommend calcium tablets in addition to milk. If you take calcium tablets, it is important to take them on an empty stomach, either between meals or before meals; calcium is dissolved only in acid, and there is little or no free acid in the stomach after one has eaten. Any carelessness in obtaining sufficient calcium may cause the expectant mother's teeth to decay and her bones to become susceptible to breaks and fractures; it can prevent her infant from having normal bone structure. On the other hand, if more calcium is ingested than the body needs, it is stored in the long bones or excreted and is, therefore, harmless.

Iron and copper are essential. The need for iron and copper is also increased by pregnancy, especially during the last 2 months. In addition to the current needs of both mother and unborn child, considerable amounts of these minerals are stored by an infant before birth. If the supply is insufficient, the infant has priority over the mother. The iron and copper requirements are particularly high in the case of twins, and any insufficiency causes the babies and mother alike to become anemic. Although adequate iron and copper can be obtained from a well-planned diet, it is

[3] Adelle Davis, *Let's Cook It Right* (New York: Harcourt, Brace and Company, 1947).

well to take tablets supplying these minerals during the last half of pregnancy. Like calcium, iron and copper can be completely absorbed into the blood only when taken on an empty stomach.

Do not underestimate the importance of iodine. Another requirement which is of paramount importance is that of iodine. If iodine is lacking during pregnancy, the result is a mentally defective infant known as a cretin. A slight lack of iodine during pregnancy can cause an infant to be mentally retarded. I recently interviewed a fine mother of above average intelligence who had a 13-year-old daughter with a mental age of 6 years and another child of 5 who was mentally so subnormal that she could not utter an understandable word. The child communicated by pointing and by uttering shrill squeals. The mother had lived in the Northwest goiter belt during both pregnancies. Although the parents had spent thousands of dollars trying to find help for the children, physicians had told them repeatedly that nothing could be done; the low intake of iodine during pregnancy was the cause. The heartbroken mother sat across from me and sobbed, and you would have cried with her as I did.

Studies of extremely large infants, the 12- and 14-pounders, have shown that such babies usually result when the mother's basal metabolism is low because of insufficient iodine intake and/or perhaps lack of B vitamins. Certainly no woman wishes to face the difficult delivery of such an infant.

Regardless of where you live, see that all the salt you eat during pregnancy is iodized salt. If your salt intake is restricted, substitute for it some other source of iodine. In case you live in the goiter belt of the Middle West or the Pacific Northwest or any other region where persons are susceptible to goiter, ask your physician about taking some reliable source of iodine such as Lugol's solution or potassium iodide tablets.

Other minerals. There are many other minerals needed in larger amounts during pregnancy, but these are generously supplied in the American diet, as are phosphorus and potassium, or are assumed to be adequately supplied. Those assumed to be supplied include the trace minerals such as magnesium, manganese, cobalt, and fluorine. Instead of recommending that calcium, iron, and iodine be taken separately, I usually advise expectant mothers to take tablets of mixed minerals which include calcium, phosphorus, iron, copper, iodine, and a number of trace minerals. Such products are available, and your obstetrician or druggist can probably help you obtain them.

Obtain adequate vitamin A. Numerous surveys of the diets of large groups of our people have shown that the average daily intake of vitamin A ranges from 1,500 to 2,000 units. Such amounts cannot meet the demands of pregnancy. Although vitamin A is widespread, an expectant mother can rarely get sufficient amounts of this nutrient from foods. She must control her weight and therefore forgo such sources as large amounts of cream and butter. She may absorb only a small amount of vitamin A (carotene) from fruits and vegetables. Dr. Eddy points out in his book *Vitaminology* [4] that only about 1 per cent of the carotene is absorbed from carrots eaten raw compared with 30 per cent when they are cooked.

About the only sources of vitamin A which are adequate in amount, readily absorbed, and practically free from calories are concentrates of fish-liver oil. These concentrates are available in capsules supplying 5,000 to 50,000 units each. I usually recommend that an expectant mother in good health take one 25,000-unit capsule daily throughout her pregnancy. Capsules of this potency cost little more than do those supplying 5,000 units; buy them for the cheapest price you can find. Since malformations are produced in the young of animals deficient in this vitamin, an adequate amount of this nutrient may be extremely important.

Carotene and vitamin A, like vitamins D, E, and K, dissolve in fat. These fat-soluble vitamins are efficiently carried into the blood only after they have combined with bile salts. When concentrates of these vitamins are used, they should be taken after meals; then a greater amount of bile flows into the intestine than at other times.

[4] W. H. Eddy, *Vitaminology* (Baltimore: The Williams and Wilkins Company, 1950).

The B vitamins are as scarce as hens' teeth. It is extremely difficult for anyone to obtain sufficient amounts of the B vitamins from our American diet. For a pregnant woman to eat enough foods supplying these vitamins to meet her ideal needs is an almost impossible task. Furthermore, the richest sources of these vitamins are foods which are little used and which most people find unpalatable. Yet to eat them is vital; most of the complications of pregnancy are caused by a lack of these vitamins.

Every scientist agrees that the requirements of the B vitamins are increased by pregnancy, but there is total disagreement as to the extent of the increase. The estimates vary from one and a half times the nonpregnant requirement to five times that amount. Dr. Tom Spies, head of the School of Nutrition at the Northwestern University College of Medicine, whose clinical work in the B vitamins has been outstanding, recommends that 5 milligrams of vitamin B_1 [5] be obtained daily. This quantity should be supplied by natural foods containing all the B vitamins, which number twelve or more.

Only three foods are excellent sources of these vitamins: wheat germ, liver, and powdered brewers' yeast. Since the B vitamins are not stored in the body, one or more of these foods should be eaten every day throughout your pregnancy. Yeast is the most concentrated source; try to take at least 1 heaping tablespoon daily and preferably 3. If yeast is new to you, start by stirring 1 teaspoon into a glass of your favorite juice and increase the amount gradually. The easiest way to prepare larger quantities is to empty a pint of juice into a wide-mouth quart jar, add 4 tablespoons of yeast, stir slightly, fill the jar with water, and set in the refrigerator; the lumps will disintegrate on standing. Stir well before using and prepare more whenever the jar is empty. Since the B vitamins are readily lost in the urine if large amounts are obtained at one time, take no more than 1 tablespoon of yeast before or between each meal.

Use wheat germ daily as a cereal or add it to cereal. Wheat

[5] R. R. Williams and T. Spies, *Vitamin B₁ in Medicine* (New York: The Macmillan Company, 1938), p. 82.

germ and middlings make a delicious cooked cereal, especially when simmered in milk. Raw wheat germ can be made palatable enough to eat alone as a cold cereal if toasted on a cookie sheet at 275 degrees F. for about 1 hour. Although some of its nutritive value is undoubtedly destroyed, more wheat germ is usually eaten when it is toasted, and therefore more vitamins are probably obtained. Use wheat germ in cooking in every way you can. Eat liver at least once each week and preferably more often.

Another possible source of B vitamins is the Bulgarian cultured milk, yogurt (p. 175). Although yogurt itself is not a rich source of these vitamins, evidence indicates that the valuable bacteria supplied by the yogurt produce B vitamins in the intestine.

Blackstrap molasses is a good source of the B vitamins not destroyed by heat. Whole-grain breads and cereals are fair sources; use them exclusively and avoid all products made of white flour. Certain foods contain individual B vitamins; skim milk is rich in vitamin B_2, salad oils in vitamin B_6, and meats in niacin. Only by eating wheat germ, yeast, liver, and possibly yogurt, however, can the need for the entire B group be met. Suggestions for purchasing wheat germ, brewers' yeast, and blackstrap molasses are given on page 261.

Wheat germ and yeast are both inexpensive sources of excellent protein. A pound of either wheat germ or brewers' yeast which should cost you no more than 25 and 80 cents, respectively, supplies approximately 200 grams of protein, or the amount you would obtain from steaks which might cost $10. Yogurt can be prepared inexpensively from powdered skim milk (p. 175). If you use these unusual foods, therefore, you can actually save money on your food budget. For example, since ½ cup of wheat germ supplies not only the protein equivalent of 4 eggs but also more vitamin E, the B vitamins, and iron, you need not use eggs if you eat the wheat germ.

In case you find it difficult to eat such foods as yogurt or wheat germ, take only tastes of them at first, then increase the amounts gradually. See rules for introducing these foods, page 262.

Caramel milk, or tigers' milk. If you have the character to do it, one way to obtain large amounts of protein and of the B vitamins is to drink a beverage which an imaginative youngster, interested in Tarzan, named tigers' milk. According to this small boy, tigers' milk was responsible for Tarzan's great strength. The name stuck.

Prepare tigers' milk by beating together:

        1 to 2 cups fresh skim milk
        ½ cup powdered skim milk
        1 to 4 h   ng tablespoons brewers' yeast
        1 to 3 teaspoons blackstrap molasses

When smooth, add the mixture to the remainder of the quart of fresh milk.

At first use only 1 tablespoon of yeast and 1 teaspoon of blackstrap; gradually increase the amount of each. Try to drink at least 2 glasses of this beverage daily and preferably more. I know a number of expectant mothers who drink an entire quart daily.

The value of tigers' milk is shown in the following table:

	Protein grams	Calcium grams	Iron mg.	Vitamin B₁ mg.	Vitamin B₂ mg.
1 quart skim milk	34	1.2	0.5	0.4	1.8
½ cup dried skim milk (100 grams)	35	1.2	0.5	0.4	1.8
4 heaping tablespoons yeast (45 grams each)	80	0.2	29.2	16.2	8.7
3 teaspoons blackstrap *	0	0.3	9.6	0.5	0.6
Total if a quart is taken daily	149	2.9	39.8	17.5	12.9

mg. = milligrams.

* Blackstrap molasses is rich in pantothenic acid, inositol, various minerals, and other nutrients not shown on the table.

Meeting your vitamin-C needs.

Your minimum vitamin-C requirement can most easily be met by drinking a glass of fresh orange or grapefruit juice daily. The amount of this vitamin in frozen or canned juices varies so widely with the methods of preparation and the length of time they have been stored that they cannot be recommended until the manufacturers state the vitamin content on the labels. Since the need for vitamin C is readily increased under numerous circumstances (pp. 38, 205, 230), obstetricians often recommend that vitamin-C tablets (ascorbic acid) of 100 milligrams each be taken in addition to the juice. When a large amount of vitamin C is taken at one time, much of it may be lost in the urine; therefore if you drink citrus juice at breakfast, it is best to take a tablet before lunch and dinner.

Vitamin C is more completely utilized and is needed in smaller amounts when taken with vitamin P, which is also found in citrus juices (p. 98). For this reason, vitamin-C tablets should not be entirely substituted for citrus fruit. Vitamin P, however, is not harmed by heat or oxidation and can be supplied by canned or frozen juice.

Obtain ample vitamin D without fail. Since vitamin D is necessary before calcium and phosphorus are efficiently absorbed into the blood and utilized in the body, it is especially important during pregnancy. Yet this vitamin is not supplied in foods in amounts sufficient to be dependable. The only dependable sources of vitamin D are fish-liver oils or vitamin-D preparations. Dr. Toverud, who has spent decades in vitamin-D research, stresses that if vitamin D is undersupplied in the mother's diet, babies are born prematurely and their skeletal development is so poor that they are particularly subject to birth injury. Furthermore, unless vitamin D is adequately supplied in the mother's diet, it is difficult to prevent the infant from developing rickets.

Although the usual recommendation for vitamin D is only 400 to 800 units daily throughout pregnancy, women taking that amount may give birth to infants with poor bone structure; the tiny facial bones are often narrow and underdeveloped, the skull elongated and the dental arch U-shaped. I recommend a minimum of 2,000 to 3,000 units daily. In fact, for years I have recommended that an expectant mother take a single capsule of 25,000 units of vitamin D each week, usually after breakfast every Sunday. As a rule these women have had easy deliveries, and invariably their infants have excellent bone structure.

The easiest and cheapest means of taking vitamin D is in capsules of 25,000 units each. Any druggist can order them for you. The vitamin can also be obtained from cod-liver-oil capsules supplying vitamin A as well; the label should be carefully read, and the dosage determined accordingly.

Although vitamin D is often added to calcium tablets or similar preparations, the vitamin is unstable when mixed with minerals. Under no circumstances should vitamin D from this source be relied upon.

Vitamin E may be essential. The amount of vitamin E needed during pregnancy has not been established. It probably is needed, however, in larger than normal amounts. Dr. Young (ref. 3, p. 17), professor of obstetrics at the University of London, points out that women obtaining too little vitamin E often develop toxemia and frequently have premature babies. Unless an expectant mother can eat ½ cup of wheat germ—the richest source of vitamin E—daily throughout her pregnancy, I recommend that she take a capsule of this vitamin supplying 30 milligrams of alpha tocopherol. Like vitamins A and D, vitamin E must be taken after meals to be efficiently absorbed.

Vitamin K can prevent lifelong tragedy. Vitamin K is necessary before blood can clot normally. Although it is generously supplied in foods and is produced by bacteria in the intestinal tract, it does not readily pass through the placenta into the unborn baby's blood. For this reason, hemorrhage in newborn infants is extremely common. Hemorrhage occurring in the brain or spinal cord of the newborn is thought to be sometimes responsible for that lifelong tragedy—spastic paralysis. Most obstetricians now give injections of vitamin K to the mother during labor and/or to the infant immediately after birth. Unfortunately such a precaution is not universal.

As a precautionary measure I recommend that an expectant

mother purchase vitamin K, which has the jaw-breaking name of 2-methyl-1-4-naphthoquinone, in 5-milligram tablets. If her infant has not arrived prematurely, she should take one daily during the last week of her pregnancy. I ask her to take a tablet every hour as soon as she notices the first signs of labor and to keep a few tablets in her purse to take on the way to the hospital. The amount she will take will probably cost no more than 10 cents; the tablets, although salty, can be taken without water; this synthetic vitamin K dissolves in water rather than fat and therefore passes quickly into the infant's blood; and the vitamin is not harmful if taken in amounts greater than needed.

Are multivitamin capsules justified? Many obstetricians recommend multivitamin capsules which supply five B vitamins rather than insisting that these vitamins be obtained from natural foods which can supply all twelve or more of them. It is better, they reason, to have the diet adequate in some B vitamins than in none.

Although I have tried dozens of varieties of these capsules, I have yet to find one which can give you that top-of-the-world feeling you can get by taking yeast.

Multivitamin capsules usually do not supply choline, for example, which may be more important during pregnancy than any other B vitamin, although a few capsules supply one-fiftieth of a day's requirement of choline. It is known that choline is efficiently used only when still another B vitamin, inositol, is obtained in adequate amounts. Such capsules do not supply the B vitamins para aminobenzoic acid, biotin, folic acid, or vitamin B_{12}; yet a deficiency of any one of these vitamins can result in the anemias which frequently occur during pregnancy. Since the B vitamins are found together in foods, a deficiency of only one of the vitamins probably never occurs.

Evidence indicates that the taking of any one or more B vitamins increases the need for all the other vitamins of the group. It may be that the B vitamins supplied in multivitamin capsules actually cause the need for such vitamins as B_{12} or choline to be increased and that taking such preparations could be a factor in bringing about anemia or toxemia during pregnancy. For this reason I consider them dangerous and not to be recommended unless foods rich in all the B vitamins are taken with them.

Your daily schedule. The following menus are suggested to show how the required nutrients may be obtained. The position of the supplements indicates which should be taken before meals and which afterward. Your daily schedule may be somewhat as follows:

BREAKFAST:

calcium and/or tablets supplying iron and copper or mixed minerals
8 ounces citrus juice or 100 milligrams vitamin C
¼ to ½ cup wheat germ with milk
1 egg and/or crisp bacon if desired
1 slice whole-wheat toast if desired
1 glass fortified milk
1 cup coffee if desired
1 vitamin-A capsule, 25,000 units
1 vitamin-E capsule, 30 milligrams, unless ½ cup of wheat germ has
   been eaten
1 vitamin-D capsule, 25,000 units, taken every Sunday unless 2,000
   to 3,000 units of the vitamin is taken daily with vitamin A

MIDMORNING:

1 heaping tablespoon yeast in 8 ounces juice or in tigers' milk
   and/or citrus fruit if not eaten at breakfast

LUNCH:

calcium and/or iron or mixed-mineral tablets
1 vitamin-C tablet, 100 milligrams
1 egg, if none for breakfast, and/or cheese or meat or cream soup
1 vegetable, raw or cooked; more if desired
1 glass fortified milk or tigers' milk
fruit or milk dessert if desired

MIDAFTERNOON:

1 heaping tablespoon yeast in 8 ounces juice or in tigers' milk or
   citrus juice if not taken earlier

DINNER:

calcium and/or iron or mixed-mineral tablets *1 tsp. lecithin in tom. juice*

✓ 1 vitamin-C tablet, 100 milligrams

soup, tomato juice, or fish or fruit cocktail if desired *190 kcal*

✓ meat, fish, or fowl, or meat substitute *4 oz.* *92 prt*

✓ 1 or 2 cooked vegetables *prt* *40 mg*

✓ salad, with cottage cheese if cheese has not been eaten at lunch *yogurt doz dress*

1 glass fortified milk or tigers' milk; more if desired *208 (126)*

✓ fruit or milk dessert *ice cream n custard and yogurt* *540*

BEFORE BED:

✓ 1 heaping tablespoon yeast in juice or tigers' milk or 1 glass fortified milk

The foregoing schedule is merely a goal to strive toward. If
the amounts of food are more than you can eat comfortably, try
to eat those which are most essential and let the others go.

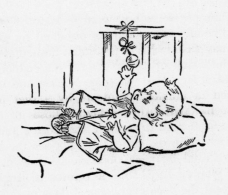

CHAPTER 4

COMPLICATIONS
DURING PREGNANCY

PREGNANCY is a normal physiological function which should proceed without any complications whatsoever. During this period, a healthy woman feels greater vigor and more joy in living than usual. Yet complications are so common that they are frequently looked upon as inevitable. Often a woman will not even report them to her obstetrician until they become so severe that he has little chance to help her. A good rule to follow is to tell your doctor about every minor deviation from health and let him evaluate it.

Nausea. Your physician will want to know if you experience nausea. Good results are sometimes obtained by glandular therapy, and he may wish to begin treatment immediately.

Although the causes of nausea are not understood, it is usually associated with a lack of B vitamins. Nausea and vomiting have been produced in human volunteers by a diet inadequate in vitamin B_1 or B_6 (pyridoxin).[1] Massive doses of both of these vitamins have been used in treating the nausea and vomiting of pregnancy, but vitamin B_6 appears to produce the better results. The procedure used by most obstetricians now is to give 100 milligrams of vitamin B_6 as soon as nausea is first noticed; they sometimes repeat the dose every 3 or 4 days or recommend that tablets supplying 10 milligrams of the vitamin be taken as frequently as are needed to control any return of nausea, often every 3 hours. Since the taking of any B vitamin can apparently increase

[1] J. E. Mueller and R. W. Vilter, "Pyridoxin Deficiency in Human Beings Induced by Desoxypyridoxine," *Journal of Clinical Investigation*, **29** (1950), 193.

the need for other vitamins of the B group, foods rich in all these vitamins should be substituted for the vitamin tablets as quickly as your tolerance for food permits. In order to prevent nausea, especially if you have suffered from it during a previous pregnancy, it is probably wise to start taking 5-milligram tablets of both B_1 and B_6 daily as soon as you find you are pregnant.

Before nausea occurs, the amount of sugar in the blood usually drops below normal. High blood sugar is maintained by a diet rich in protein. The reason nausea is most often experienced in the early morning is that a woman has not eaten during the night and her blood sugar is lowest at this time. Just before you retire, eat food containing both protein and natural sugar or starch, which is changed into sugar. Keep a plate of cheese and whole-wheat crackers or other nutritious food by your bedside and eat during the night if you should awake; eat again 15 to 30 minutes before getting up.

In case you lose meals or fail to eat frequently, a condition known as acetone acidosis occurs. A somewhat toxic substance, acetone, accumulates in your blood, and although it is gradually thrown off in your breath and urine, it can cause headache and further nausea. Studies have shown, however, that acetone is detoxified by vitamin C. Before nausea becomes a problem, therefore, it is well to take 100 milligrams of this vitamin with each meal. In case nausea develops to the point of your losing meals, take 5 to 10 tablets of vitamin C, 100 milligrams each, before going to bed, the amount depending on the degree of nausea experienced.

Often vomiting starts because women who have not felt like eating become starved and overeat; chances are the meal is lost a few minutes later. Since an upset stomach cannot tolerate being overloaded, such folly should be carefully avoided. Eat something every 2 hours throughout the entire day. Instead of having a breakfast of fruit juice, cereal, egg, toast, and coffee, have only the egg, toast, and coffee; 2 hours later drink the juice, and after another interval eat the cereal or the equivalent in milk and whole-wheat bread or crackers. Follow the same procedure with lunch and dinner. It may be a nuisance but will pay dividends.

Since nausea occurs at the period when malnutrition can impose such a severe penalty, do your best to eat foods which are the most essential. On the other hand, avoid nutritious foods if they are particularly repulsive to you, and try to find a substitute. I have known women so eager to have healthy babies that they have made themselves drink milk or eat liver, wheat germ, or yeast at this time even though they had always disliked these foods; then they became so ill that they could not tolerate such foods during the remainder of their pregnancy. In such a case it is better to take calcium tablets and vitamin-B-complex capsules, however inadequate they may be, until you can drink milk or eat foods naturally rich in the B vitamins without feeling squeamish.

During severe nausea you can protect the embryo by taking vitamins and minerals in tablet or capsule form. Follow the general suggestions on page 35, but take them at the time when you are least nauseated. Since so many foods contain protein, you can surely find a few which appeal to your appetite. Count the grams of protein you obtain daily (p. 24), and try to meet your requirement as nearly as possible.

Threatened miscarriage. If you show spotting, call your obstetrician immediately. In case you cannot reach him, stay in bed until you can.

Adequate nutrition prior to conception probably plays an important role in preventing miscarriage. Whether nutrition can help to prevent a threatened miscarriage is not known. A safe rule is to eat the best diet you can in the hope that it will help. Vitamin E has at times appeared to be of particular value. For example, women with threatened miscarriage have been given 30 milligrams of vitamin E, or alpha tocopherol, daily; 90 per cent of them carried through their pregnancies successfully.[2] Other physicians have found that vitamin-E therapy does not help at all.

[2] Franklin Bicknell and Frederick Prescott, *The Vitamins in Medicine* (2d ed.; London: Heinemann Medical Books, Ltd., 1948), p. 746.

Studies of the embryos of women who have miscarried show that a large per cent are so defective that, if the pregnancy had continued, malformed children might have resulted. Such research has caused many obstetricians to feel that a miscarriage is nature's method of maintaining high standards. If such be the case, it may be well to allow nature to take its own course. The best diet possible should be followed, however, in case the pregnancy continues. If the pregnancy is terminated, such a diet should be followed in preparation for a later conception.

Fatigue. Another problem which frequently arises during pregnancy is that of fatigue. The most common cause of fatigue due to poor nutrition is a deficiency of protein, which is essential in keeping the blood sugar high, and lack of B vitamins (p. 29), which are necessary before energy can be produced. The fatigue which occurs before meals, as in the late morning and afternoon, is generally caused by a decrease in blood sugar; it can be readily corrected by eating meals high in protein (ref. 2, p. 108) and taking between meals some foods containing natural sugar or unrefined starch. Early morning fatigue is most often associated with low blood pressure and disappears as soon as the blood pressure is brought up to normal (p. 50). Fatigue which is persistent throughout the day is usually caused by anemia (p. 50). If you find yourself with too little energy, eat liver every day until you feel better, in addition to taking perhaps ½ cup of wheat germ daily and drinking 2 or 3 tablespoons of yeast in fruit juice between meals. Often a pickup can be noticed after a single day.

Nervous tension, insomnia, and leg cramps. Other symptoms which are often intensified during pregnancy are a tendency to become more high-strung, inability to sleep soundly, and perhaps cramps in the calves of the legs, particularly during the night. These abnormalities occur when calcium is undersupplied or is poorly absorbed. Leg cramps, however, caused by muscular strain as a woman becomes heavier and leans backward to balance her center of gravity, can also occur even when the diet is amply supplied with calcium.

If you drink daily 1 quart of skim milk fortified with powdered milk, and if you take calcium tablets before meals, the nervousness, insomnia, and leg cramps resulting from calcium deficiency will probably soon disappear. When sleeplessness and nocturnal leg cramps are problems, it is often wise to take calcium tablets just before retiring; keep the tablets by the bedside and take more during the night if wakeful or if the leg cramps recur.

Heartburn and gas distention, or flatulence. The requirements of the B vitamins are so difficult to meet during pregnancy that heartburn and gas distention often result from the undersupply of these nutrients. Heartburn is caused by gases escaping upward from the stomach with sufficient force to push a small amount of hydrochloric acid before them; the strong acid irritates the delicate lining of the esophagus. The gases may come from the fermentation of foods in the intestine or may be merely swallowed air. Large amounts of air are swallowed when one eats rapidly or gulps liquid. A tense, high-strung person swallows air almost continuously. Such a person usually relaxes, and air swallowing ceases to be a problem, when the diet is made adequate in calcium, vitamin D, and all the B vitamins. Much air gulping can be prevented if straws are used temporarily for drinking all cold liquids.

Avoid taking baking soda to relieve heartburn at any time during pregnancy, particularly if your obstetrician asks you to limit your salt intake. In such a case, he wants you to obtain less sodium; baking soda is almost pure sodium and can be dangerous if certain complications of pregnancy should arise.

Whenever foods are incompletely digested, large amounts of gas are formed by bacteria in the intestine. If the B vitamins are undersupplied, the flow of digestive juices and the production of digestive enzymes decrease; the movements of the intestine slow down so that undigested food is not brought into contact with enzymes; the digested food is not carried to the intestinal wall where it can pass into the blood. Hence much undigested food remains in the large intestine to support the growth of millions of bacteria.

If a person suffering from gas pain or distention improves his diet by eating wheat germ or yeast, part of the food is digested, and some of the vitamins are absorbed. A portion of the food, however, usually remains undigested. Since bacteria require B vitamins, and since the more B vitamins supplied them, the more rapidly they multiply, they thrive on their improved diet, and the amount of gas formed is often greatly increased. In this case it is wise to eat only a small amount of foods rich in B vitamins at one time so that it can be completely digested; perhaps 1 tablespoon of wheat germ could be eaten at each meal and 1 teaspoon of yeast in juice or milk sipped every 2 hours.

Whenever gas is a problem, it is wise to take tablets of digestive enzyme after meals for a few days, or until the body is supplied with enough B vitamins to produce a normal amount of enzymes. Such tablets are available at drugstores. The trouble with recommending digestive enzymes is that a person taking them often gets such marked relief that he does not want to give them up even when he no longer needs them.

Constipation and hemorrhoids. Since the B vitamins are necessary before energy can be produced normally, a lack of these vitamins causes a slowing down throughout the body. Too little motility in the large intestine allows the waste material to remain overlong and to become hard and dry; constipation is the result. Any good source of B vitamins, therefore, is laxative, whether liver, wheat germ, brewers' yeast, or blackstrap molasses. Of the four, blackstrap is probably the most laxative. Stools usually become soft and elimination regular within 3 or 4 days after generous amounts of these foods are eaten. During the last months of pregnancy, when the enlarged uterus presses against the rectum, constipation may result unless large amounts of foods rich in B vitamins are consumed daily.

When the constipation is unusually stubborn, certain temporary procedures can be followed. For example, if yogurt (p. 175) is eaten at each meal with 1 teaspoon of milk sugar sprinkled over it, the stools invariably become soft and bulky. The bacteria of the yogurt live on the milk sugar and form tiny bubbles of gas throughout the waste material, causing it to have the texture of a loaf of bread ready to be put into an oven. Another temporary measure is to take tablets of dried bile, which is laxative, at each meal; tablets of bile mixed with laxatives, however, should be avoided.

All laxatives and cathartics are harmful in some way. They push food through the digestive tract ahead of schedule, thus interfering with digestion and absorption by cutting down the time the food mass remains in the small intestine; many laxatives interfere with absorption and may cause dehydration by attracting water from the blood into the intestine; others irritate the delicate linings of the intestine and cause them to "weep" much as something in your eye will stimulate the flow of tears. Studies have shown that the bulk-forming laxatives, thought to be harmless, mechanically interfere with both the digestion and absorption of nutrients. When enemas are used, the water forced against delicate membranes is rarely sterile, mucus which protects the lining of the colon is washed away, and tiny muscles surrounding the rectum are often broken. Mineral oil is perhaps the most dangerous of all laxatives. When mineral oil is taken internally, carotene and vitamins A, D, E, and K in the blood and body tissues readily dissolve in it and are then excreted; thus mineral oil may produce harmful deficiencies in both you and your unborn baby.

Hemorrhoids are bits of tissue from the lining of the rectum pushed through the anus by mechanical means. Either the passing of hard, dry stools or the quick, forceful evacuations which result from the use of cathartics can cause such injury. When the stools are kept soft by a diet rich in B vitamins, and when cathartics and laxatives are avoided, hemorrhoids can be prevented and those which already exist usually disappear.

Neuritis. Few complications of pregnancy have been studied so thoroughly as has neuritis, which results when vitamin B₁ is undersupplied. Usually neuritis is corrected as soon as this vitamin is added generously to the diet. Neuritis starts with fatigue and an "all-gone" feeling. Recurring numbness and vague, fleeting pains may be felt in the hands, feet, and shoulders. The hands and feet "go to sleep" easily, and a prickling needles-and-pins sensation is often noticed. As neuritis becomes more severe, steady pain follows the nerve channels and may become excruciating indeed.

Physicians usually treat neuritis by giving injections of vitamin B_1, which often brings immediate relief. Since much of the vitamin is lost in the urine within a few hours, however, the pain may soon recur. In addition to the injections, many obstetricians advise their patients to take 5-milligram tablets of vitamin B_1 by mouth every 2 or 3 hours—the frequency depending upon the severity of the pain—until the neuritis disappears. Research has consistently shown that better results are obtained when foods rich in all the B vitamins are eaten in addition to the taking of vitamin-B_1 injections or tablets.

Such complications as anemia, low and high blood pressure, swollen ankles and albumin in the urine are discussed in the following chapter.

Most of the complications of pregnancy are related in one way or another to a diet which is not completely adequate. The expectant mother herself usually determines whether she will suffer from few complications or many and whether they will be mild or severe.

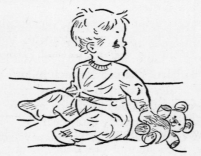

CHAPTER 5

RECOGNIZE THE DANGER WARNINGS

"SOME women just won't follow a diet," Dr. Williams remarked to me one day.

I might have disagreed with him if it had not been for Margaret. She was thrilled to be pregnant again; her boy was almost 14, her girl about 9, and both were lovely children. I knew she was not eating correctly, and more than once I tried to get her to improve her diet.

"Phooey on that stuff," she would answer gaily. "I have two beautiful children, and I didn't eat a bunch of junk when I was pregnant with them."

"Are you taking the vitamin capsules and mineral tablets your doctor recommended?" I asked her.

"I intend to, but I can't remember them. But I've been watching my weight. Been living on cucumbers; they're so good now. Of course I go to a lot of parties. Such food! Far be it from me ever to insult a hostess."

When the danger signals appeared, her obstetrician and I both talked turkey to her, but our arguments fell on deaf ears. She laughingly told me her doctor had said, "When you shuffle a deck of cards, the aces don't always fall on top."

In her seventh month she developed eclampsia. Her baby was born dead, and she was frightfully ill. Her obstetrician—a grand person—felt that he had failed; yet it was not his fault. If she had known more about nutrition and had understood something of the physiology of pregnancy, such a tragedy could have been prevented.

The responsibility is the expectant mother's. At the Chicago Lying-in Hospital the cornerstone of every building except one bears the name of some great physician who has made an outstanding contribution in the field of obstetrics. One cornerstone has been reserved for the name of the person who discovers the cause of toxemia; that cornerstone is still bare. As in Margaret's case, the symptoms of this condition seem insignificant to thousands of expectant mothers. To obstetricians—and a finer group of men I have yet to meet—these same symptoms cause dread and fear. From the first day you report to your obstetrician, he is on the lookout for these symptoms and tries to prevent them. It is for this reason he asks you to visit him each month or more often and to bring a urine sample each time; it is for this reason he checks your blood pressure and watches your weight fluctuations so carefully. And more than one obstetrician, after trying desperately and staying calm and efficient until everything has been done which could be done, has sobbed like a child and blamed himself because he was unable to save the infant or to prevent the mother's death.

It seems to me that these fine men have been blaming themselves for something for which they are not to blame. They have shouldered a responsibility which has been impossible for them to fulfill for two reasons: first, because until recently there has been no inkling of what factors allowed toxemia to develop; and second, because they, like Margaret's doctor, cannot go home with each patient and do her eating for her.

It now appears that toxemia develops only when certain nutritional deficiencies exist. As I see it, the expectant mother (and she alone) can prevent this dreaded condition. It may seem to some that the material in this chapter is of a medical nature which should be left to the obstetricians. Until an expectant mother learns, however, that seemingly insignificant symptoms can change with lightning speed into dangerous ones, and until she knows how nutritional deficiencies can be overcome, she cannot take steps to prevent or to correct these symptoms. Until then obstetricians will continue to blame themselves. In case you develop the danger warnings mentioned in this chapter, by all means discuss them with your obstetrician, but keep the responsibility of correcting them on your own shoulders.

The most serious complication of pregnancy. The most dangerous complication of pregnancy is toxemia, or pre-eclampsia, which can develop into the even more serious condition, eclampsia. Toxemia literally means toxins in the blood. Since no toxins may be present, the medical term pre-eclampsia is more accurate. I shall, however, use the word toxemia because it is probably more familiar to you.

Toxemia is responsible for the majority of stillborn babies, for approximately 50 per cent of all premature births, and, when it develops into eclampsia, for one-fifth of all maternal deaths. During the past few decades, deaths of infants under 1 year old have decreased tremendously. Deaths of infants under 1 month, however, have not decreased; in fact, many investigations indicate that they have increased. The majority of infants who die during the first month of life are those who have been born prematurely, or whose mothers in more than half the cases have suffered from toxemia.

In case eclampsia develops, birth must usually be induced to save the mother; if other attempts should be unsuccessful, a Caesarean section must be performed. Even if all goes well with both mother and infant, the cost of the delivery has probably doubled, the mother's convalescence is considerably lengthened, her chances of nursing her baby are practically nil, and any babies she may have in the future must also be delivered by Caesarean section.

At a recent public health meeting in our city, the head nurse of one of the large hospitals stressed the fact that during the past 2 years there had been a tremendous increase in the incidence of toxemia and in the number of infants who were being born prematurely. She further stated that though no one knew the cause, we would be glad to know that the hospital had opened new wards and trained special staffs for the purpose of caring for these premature infants. Any person with a knowledge of nutrition would have guessed the cause to be the high price of food which often made it impossible for expectant mothers to obtain an adequate diet.

The symptoms of toxemia. Most obstetricians consider toxemia to be any case in which the blood pressure is above 140/90 or in which a moderate to large amount of albumin is excreted in the urine. The onset of toxemia is characterized by a sudden increase in blood pressure. One case cited in the medical literature was that of a woman whose blood pressure had been 90/60 one week but had shot up to 179/110 by the following week. There is often a rapid gain in weight caused by pounds of water being held in the body, a condition known as edema. The most common symptom noticed by the woman herself is that of swollen ankles, although she may also suffer from headache, pain above her stomach, and visual disturbances. If the condition becomes worse, the mother develops convulsions, and usually the pregnancy must be terminated.

Toxemia can be prevented. Obstetricians by no means agree that the cause or causes of toxemia are known. Toxemia, however, has been repeatedly produced in experimental animals.[1,2] It would appear from the research that toxemia can result from separate or combined deficiencies of the B vitamins, particularly choline, and of protein, especially of the amino acid, methionine.

Few studies appear to have been made of pregnant women whose diets have been adequate in protein and all the B vitamins. In a study of 1,400 cases, however, Dr. Holmes[3] compared the incidence of toxemia among women eating varying amounts of protein. He found that expectant mothers who ate 60 to 70 grams of protein daily suffered from toxemia almost twice as much as did another group having a daily intake of 110 to 120 grams of protein. Similarly, in a study made at Philadelphia General

[1] K. Schwarz, "Rat Eclampsia, a Deficiency Disease of Dual Origin," *Nutrition Abstracts and Reviews*, 3678, **19** (1950), 3.

[2] W. E. Armstrong and P. P. Swanson, "A Syndrome of Dietary Origin in the Pregnant Rat Resembling Toxemia in Pregnancy," *American Journal of the Dietetics Association*, **19** (1943), 756.

[3] O. M. Holmes, "Protein Diet in Pregnancy," *Western Journal of Surgery, Obstetrics, and Gynecology*, **49** (1941), 57.

Hospital,[4] it was found that when women ate so little protein that the amount of protein in their blood dropped below normal, 26 per cent of them developed toxemia. When the women were classified according to the amounts of protein in their blood, those showing the lowest blood protein had a much higher percentage of toxemia than did those whose blood proteins were more nearly normal.

Another study was made of over 5,000 women coming into the prenatal clinics of ten London hospitals.[5] A detailed survey of the food eaten by these women showed that their diets were grossly inadequate in almost every respect. The women were then divided into two groups; the women of one group remained on their usual diet, whereas the others were given supplements, donated by pharmaceutical firms, of iron, calcium, vitamins A, C, D, and all the B vitamins. Despite the fact that the protein intake was low, the women whose diets were supplemented suffered far less from toxemia and had fewer premature and stillborn infants than did the women who received no supplements.

It is frequently pointed out that a much higher incidence of toxemia occurs among women who come to free prenatal clinics than among those seen by an obstetrician in his private practice. Women who go to free clinics can rarely afford good diets rich in expensive proteins; they usually are unaware of the value of nutrition. The physicians who give their time to such clinics are too swamped with work to make out individual diet plans. The women going to private physicians can afford better diets, have more knowledge of nutrition, and are usually given diet lists to guide them.

In Europe during both world wars, the incidence of toxemia markedly decreased. Sugar became unavailable, and jams, jellies, pastries, and desserts were no longer eaten. In most countries the complete milling of grains was prohibited, and only whole-

[4] J. D. Bibb, "Protein and Hemoglobin in Normal and Toxic Pregnancies," *Am. J. Obst. Gynec.*, 42 (1941), 103.

[5] Interim Report of the Peoples League of Health: Nutrition of Expectant and Nursing Mothers, *Lancet*, 2 (1942), 10.

grain breads and cereals were allowed. Since little other food was to be had, the consumption of breadstuffs increased. The B vitamins, vitamin E, and the valuable protein of the wheat germ, so badly needed by expectant mothers, were supplied.

Certainly toxemia does not occur without first giving ample warning. Let us see what the danger signals are and learn how to correct them as soon as they first appear.

Anemia can be a warning. Anemia, so prevalent during pregnancy, is usually assumed to be caused merely by lack of iron, as indeed it sometimes is. Anemia can be produced in experimental animals by diets lacking in only one of several B vitamins: vitamin B_1, or thiamin; vitamin B_6, or pyridoxin; niacin; folic acid; biotin; choline; or vitamin B_{12}. This disease has also been produced in human volunteers by diets inadequate in most of these vitamins. Two forms of anemia common during the last of pregnancy are unaffected by iron, but one is corrected by the B vitamin, choline, and the other form, by folic acid and vitamin B_{12}.

Anemia also occurs when the diet is inadequate in protein. Dr. Bibb (ref. 4, p. 49) of the Philadelphia General Hospital, studied anemia in a large group of expectant mothers all of whom had been given the same amount of iron. The women whose blood proteins were low had anemia, and those who had normal blood protein did not. Furthermore, his study showed that the anemia paralleled the incidence of toxemia.

If you are anemic during your pregnancy, take tablets supplying iron, but do not be content until your supply of B vitamins and proteins has been increased. The anemia can be a warning that toxemia may be expected. If you enjoy liver, the best way to correct anemia is to have a serving of liver daily for 2 or 3 weeks. Dip the liver in wheat germ and sauté it lightly. Liver supplies not only iron but protein of excellent quality and all the B vitamins, and is rich in both methionine and choline.

Beware of low blood pressure. Many women, realizing that high blood pressure can be dangerous during pregnancy, actually feel safe when they learn that their blood pressure is below normal. Such a feeling of security is extremely false; low blood pressure can change to high blood pressure with startling rapidity (p. 48). Low blood pressure can be produced experimentally by diets low in either protein or the B vitamins, the very nutrients which appear to be important in preventing toxemia.

When the diet is made adequate, low blood pressure usually becomes normal within 1 or 2 weeks. As soon as the pressure increases, the tissues receive more nourishment; hence the woman experiences a feeling of well-being and a marked pickup in energy.

Watch for swollen ankles. If your ankles start to swell, you may be eating too little protein or losing it in the urine. Swollen ankles, though by no means confined to expectant mothers, are particularly common during pregnancy because the protein requirements are markedly increased.

Under normal circumstances, a certain amount of a protein, albumin, is found in the blood. As the blood leaves the arteries and passes through the capillary beds, each heartbeat forces blood plasma into the tissues; eventually almost nothing is left in the capillaries except red blood corpuscles and blood proteins. At this point the albumin serves its purpose by attracting back into the blood the fluids from the cells carrying waste products. These waste products are then removed by the kidneys.

Before the body can maintain a normal amount of albumin in the blood, adequate protein of high quality must be eaten. If protein or even one amino acid, such as methionine, is supplied in too small a quantity, little albumin can be formed, and the amount in the blood decreases. Consequently fluids containing waste products cannot be efficiently drawn into the blood; some remain in the tissues. Such a condition is spoken of as edema. Because of gravity, edema is first noticeable in the ankles of a person who is standing or walking a good deal; but after a night's rest the ankles are usually normal in size, whereas the fingers and eyes are often puffy. Dr. Spitzer,[6] who has studied

---

[6] H. Spitzer, "Protein Depletion in Pregnancy Toxemia," *West. J. Surg., Obst., Gynec.,* **54** (1946), 392.

the amount of protein in the blood of women suffering from toxemia, suggests that it is the waste-contaminated fluids held in the brain which cause the convulsions of eclampsia.

I recently saw a woman whose ankles were extremely swollen, although she was in only her fourth month of pregnancy. She was eating little protein and was not drinking milk because she feared she would gain too much. Within 3 days after she increased her protein intake, the swelling disappeared. What pleased her even more, the scales showed she had lost 6 pounds; such a loss meant that some 3 quarts of liquid had been held in her tissues.

If your ankles start to swell, count the grams of protein (pp. 24, 278) you eat. Try to get at least 150 grams or more every day until the swelling is gone. If, when your ankles swell, you do not increase the protein in your diet, realize that many pounds of waste-laden fluid are being held in your body; that your unborn baby is being affected by your impure bloodstream and is not getting the proteins needed for development; that your body lacks the proteins necessary for normal maintenance; and that serious trouble may lie ahead.

High blood pressure. Much research must be done before the high blood pressure of toxemia is understood. At the present time, its cause is unknown. High blood pressure, however, has been produced in animals by diets deficient in the B vitamin, choline. It is known that choline is more effective when given with another B vitamin, inositol, and that smaller amounts of choline are needed when the amino acid, methionine, is generously supplied. Furthermore, certain cases of high blood pressure have been successfully treated by giving both choline and inositol. The fact that the high blood pressure of pregnancy usually drops to normal after delivery indicates that its cause may be the undersupply of nutrients needed in larger amounts before the baby is born.

In case your blood pressure becomes high during pregnancy, eat as many foods rich in protein and the B vitamins as you possibly can: liver, yeast, and wheat germ. Since brain is the richest source of choline, eat it if you can endure it. Blackstrap molasses supplies so much inositol that you should take 2 or 3 tablespoons daily regardless of the fact that you may gain a few extra pounds.

When mothers suffer from high blood pressure and swollen ankles simultaneously, I ask them to take 1 rounded teaspoon of soybean lecithin in tomato juice at each meal. This product, which is available at health-food stores, is not unpalatable; yet it contains more than 30 per cent choline. As a rule the blood pressure drops and weight losses of 3 to 6 pounds occur within 1 or 2 weeks after it is taken.

Albumin in the urine. Even when women have no kidney disease, they frequently lose albumin in the urine during the last of pregnancy. Why the kidneys become so damaged that albumin, which occurs in rather large particles, can pass through them is not understood. Similar kidney damage, however, is produced experimentally when the B vitamin, choline, is undersupplied.

If albumin is found in your urine, you must be doubly careful to obtain a diet high in protein. The lost albumin comes from the blood and is badly needed to collect wastes from the tissues. If you eat sufficient protein, your liver can continuously produce albumin to replace that lost; then your ankles will not swell. Methionine, however, is necessary before albumin can be formed.

If you and your unborn baby are not to be harmed, your diet now must supply enough protein for your own needs, for your baby's growth, and *for the replacement of the albumin lost through the kidneys.* Your protein intake should probably be no less than 150 grams daily or even more if much albumin is being excreted. Select the proteins which supply the most methionine and choline (p. 57). Even though you may not enjoy these foods, realize that both your health and your baby's welfare are threatened. In comparison, surely the flavor of foods is of little importance.

Low protein diet during pregnancy. Years ago, before the mechanism of urine collection was understood, it was assumed that if albumin was lost in the urine, too much protein was being eaten, and the albumin was being thrown off as a waste product. Even though such reasoning was proved wrong more than 20 years ago, one still finds an obstetrician now and then who asks his patients to stay on a low protein diet. The welfare of such patients and the lives of their infants are in the laps of the gods.

I asked an obstetrician what he thought of physicians who recommended low protein diets during pregnancy. He laughed and answered, "Such men think they are practicing in 1910."

Is a diet low in salt justified? I frequently find expectant mothers who are avoiding salt even though their obstetricians have not asked them to. Salt is sodium and chlorine, both essential to health. These minerals are extremely important in keeping the body fluids neutral (from becoming either acid or alkaline). Sodium is also essential in maintaining water balance in the body. Sodium and chlorine are excreted daily in the urine, not in the form of table salt but in combination with waste products; the sodium is usually combined with uric acid (sodium urate), and the chlorine with ammonia (ammonium chloride). During pregnancy, both acid and alkaline waste products from the fetus are being thrown into the mother's blood, and her need for salt is thus increased rather than decreased.

Dr. Strauss,[7] when teaching obstetrics at Harvard Medical School, found in studying a group of women suffering from toxemia that if patients whose blood protein was low followed a diet containing large amounts of protein and as much salt as they desired, their blood pressure decreased and they lost weight, or pounds of water from their tissues. When salt was given to patients whose blood albumin was normal, even though the blood pressure was high and they suffered from other symptoms of toxemia, there was no change except a small, temporary increase in water weight. When a low protein diet and salt or baking soda (sodium bicarbonate) were given to women whose blood pressure was high, they gained water weight, the swelling

[7] M. B. Strauss, "Observations on the Etiology of the Toxemias of Pregnancy," *American Journal of Medical Science*, **194** (1937), 772.

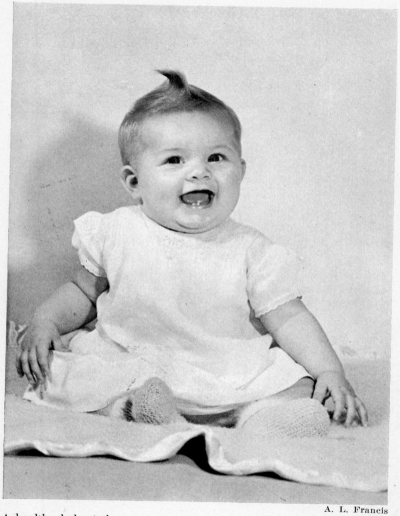

A healthy baby is happy, cries surprisingly little, and is easy to care for.

of their ankles (edema) became visibly worse, and their blood pressure increased.

Such a study indicates that salt remains in the tissues for the same reason that fluid and waste products remain there: the blood albumin is so low that these products cannot be drawn from the tissues and carried to the kidneys. At such a time both sodium and chlorine are needed to prevent the acid and alkaline waste products from harming the tissues. The important point is to increase your protein intake immediately so that sufficient albumin can be formed and all waste products can be withdrawn from the tissues.

There are times when salt, or sodium in all forms, should be avoided. For example, kidneys may be so damaged that no salt is excreted. By all means, forgo salt if your physician asks you to. To avoid it of your own accord in order to prevent swollen ankles, however, is to ignore the warning that unless your protein intake is increased, serious trouble may lie ahead.

Newer treatments of toxemia. When animals are put on a diet lacking the B vitamin, choline, the kidneys are harmed and high blood pressure is produced. When the choline-deficient diet is also limited in protein, anemia and edema, or water retention, result.[8] If the protein is increased or if only the amino acid methionine is given, the anemia and swelling are prevented or corrected. Furthermore, when young rats are given a diet lacking choline, they die of fatty livers and hemorrhages in the kidneys. Autopsies on premature infants whose mothers suffered from toxemia show similar fatty livers and kidney hemorrhages, indicating that their deaths may have been caused by deficiencies of choline.

These symptoms in animals are strikingly similar to the symptoms of toxemia. Such findings suggest that choline and methionine may be particularly important in preventing or correcting the toxemia of pregnancy.

[8] "Anemia and Edema in Chronic Choline Deficiency," *Nutrition Rev.,* **7** (1949), 298.

Dr. Strauss [9] studied a group of women suffering from non-convulsive toxemia with edema, or water retention; he gave them a diet containing 260 grams of protein daily, including almost ¾ pound of liver, rich in both choline and methionine. Almost immediately the women lost pounds of weight, showing that urine collection was again taking place normally. In no case did the blood pressure or the amount of albumin in the urine increase. None of the infants was stillborn or died soon after birth.

A similar study was made by a group of obstetricians from the McGill University Medical School.[10] At the Royal Victoria Hospital where they worked, eclampsia was responsible for a large percentage of both maternal and infant deaths. These doctors put a group of patients whom they describe as severely toxic on a diet of 110 grams of protein daily. In addition they gave the women 5 to 10 grams of methionine * daily in tablets or in powder form added to tomato juice or in intravenous injections. With the exception of one patient who died of eclampsia, all the women were markedly benefited. The edema disappeared, urine excretion became normal, and pounds of weight were lost often within a few hours after the methionine was given.

Dr. Philpott and his associates recommend that an expectant mother obtain daily at least 5 grams (5,000 milligrams) of methionine. In his book, *Vitaminology,* Dr. Eddy (ref. 4, p. 28) states that the daily requirement of choline for an adult (nonpregnant) is also 5 grams. I would venture to guess that neither of these doctors could plan a diet which contained 5,000 milligrams of each of these nutrients and still keep the quantity of food small enough for anyone to eat it.

The following table lists the richest sources of these nutrients in the amounts of foods an expectant mother might be able to take daily for a short time until any danger warning disappeared.

[9] M. B. Strauss, "Nutritional Deficiency and Water Retention in the Toxemias of Pregnancy," *J. Clin. Invest.,* 14 (1935), 710.

[10] N. W. Philpott, M. Hendelman and T. Primrose, "The Use of Methionine in Obstetrics," *Am. J. Obst. Gynec.,* 57 (1949), 125.

* Supplied by Ayerst, McKenna, and Harrison Company.

Foods to Eat Daily	Methionine * mg.	Choline † mg.	Protein grams
1 quart skim milk	930	160	34
½ cup powdered skim milk (100 grams)	930	160	35
1 egg, cooked until firm	225	280	6
½ cup cottage cheese	900 ‡	150 ‡	20
½ cup wheat germ	570	400	24
1 serving meat	580 §	90 §	15-22
or liver (¼ pound)	527	480-700	20
2 heaping tablespoons brewers' yeast (45 grams each)	1,011 ‖	360 ‖	40
2 servings cooked vegetables	0	10-300	0
Total including liver instead of other meat	5,093	2,030-2,540	181

mg. = milligrams.

* Values for methionine calculated from tables in *The Amino Acid Content of Proteins* by R. J. Block and D. Bolling (Springfield, Illinois: Charles C. Thomas and Co., 1945), pp. 209-306.

† Values for choline taken or calculated from R. W. Engle, *J. Nutrition*, **25** (1943), 441.

‡ Calculated from figures available for skim milk; some choline may be lost in the whey during cheese making.

§ Figures for beef.

‖ Calculated from analysis supplied by Anheuser Busch and Company, St. Louis, Mo., and are for their Strain G Yeast.

Even with such a diet, the choline intake is still deficient. The deficiency might be supplied by eating brains daily. The easiest method, however, is to take 1 teaspoon of soybean lecithin (p. 53) in tomato juice with each meal; 3 teaspoons of this food would supply approximately 2,000 milligrams of choline.

The warnings may seem insignificant. Almost every week I meet some pregnant woman who has two or more symptoms of impending toxemia but is unconcerned and unworried. Perhaps her ankles have been swollen now and then. Perhaps her obstetrician has told her that she is anemic or has high or low blood pressure or is losing albumin in her urine. Though she does not feel well, she thinks that is to be expected. Often she has gained 2 or 3 pounds during a week when she has eaten little; since she may know nothing of water retention, she tells herself that she must diet more carefully. At the very time when her life and that of her baby may depend upon the amount of B vitamins and proteins she obtains, she may restrict her diet until these nutrients are almost lacking. Since she may never have heard of toxemia or eclampsia or the means of preventing either, her attitudes are understandable but nevertheless heartbreaking.

Because sound nutrition is not applied, and because such symptoms seem so insignificant that they can be ignored, thousands of women give birth to full-term babies who are in far poorer physical condition than they should be. Thousands of other women have premature babies, often so weak that they die within the first month. Thousands of other women, many of whom want a child more than anything else in the world, give birth to stillborn infants.

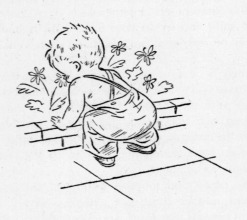

CHAPTER 6

CONTROL YOUR WEIGHT WISELY

A YOUNG woman whose mother has been a friend of mine for years dropped in on an errand. She was in her fifth month of pregnancy, and I asked her how she was getting along.

"My doctor says I'm gaining too much," she answered. "I'm so hungry all the time I'm about to die."

A comment of sympathy caused her to break into uncontrollable sobbing. I left the room and came back with a glass of skim milk. She shook her head.

"I mustn't drink it," she said. "I'm not eating between meals, and besides I've had all the milk I'm allowed for the day."

My blood began to boil. "No obstetrician on earth would expect you to suffer that much. Furthermore, your baby needs the nutrients in milk and so do you. Skim milk is one food which should never be restricted on a prenatal diet. What's more, the first law of weight control is to eat something between meals so that you won't be starved enough to overeat at the next meal."

Such a case is not unusual. One hears expectant mothers exclaim over and over again, "I'm gaining too much." There is nothing wrong with eliminating high-calorie foods which cannot build health. In order to control weight, however, it is definitely wrong to forgo low-calorie foods needed by both you and your unborn infant.

Years ago, obstetrical journals published the argument that the expectant mother must not gain excessively because her infant might become too large and her delivery more difficult. As was shown in the Harvard and Toronto studies, however, puny, poorly developed infants are difficult to deliver because the mothers of such babies are themselves in bad condition. If the mother is undernourished to the extent that water is retained in her tissues, puffy, swollen membranes actually cause the birth passage to be smaller. Furthermore, following both world wars it was found that in countries experiencing starvation, the weight of babies was approximately the same as that of infants born when food was plentiful. If the mothers were so starved that their infants were smaller, a large proportion of the babies were born dead; also great numbers of the mothers died because they did not have the reserve necessary to survive infections, hemorrhages, and shock occurring during or after their deliveries.

Of the many studies made of the factors controlling the size of the infant at birth, the only finding of significance is that the physique of the father is closely correlated to the length and weight of the baby. If you wish to have babies which are small at birth, you should marry a jockey.

Dr. King,[1] an obstetrician in Cincinnati, points out in an excellent paper that, even though it is now recognized a small baby does not assure an easy delivery nor starvation assure a small baby, the recommendation of low-calorie prenatal diets is again in vogue. The claims this time are that if weight is limited, there are fewer instances of toxemia, miscarriage, premature birth, stillbirth, malformation, and death soon after birth. These arguments Dr. King questions as being unproved and unscientific. He grants, of course, that there is an excessive weight gain at the onset of toxemia, but argues that such a gain is caused, not by a gain of fat, but by pounds of water held in the tissues. This physician holds that the only real argument against gaining too much is that the extra pounds will cause the expectant mother to be more uncomfortable during the last of her pregnancy and to be less attractive after her baby is born.

To test the claims which he considers unfounded, Dr. King made a study of 226 women whom he allowed to eat as many

[1] A. G. King, "Free-Feeding Pregnant Women," *Am. J. Obst. Gynec.*, 58 (1949), 299.

calories as they desired. He asked, however, that they take multi-vitamin capsules, calcium tablets, and, in some cases, supplements of iron. In a few instances, he requested that salt be limited but nothing else.

None of the women miscarried or developed toxemia. There were no stillbirths, and no infant was born malformed. A few of the babies were born prematurely, and three died during delivery because of complications unrelated to the weight of the mother, such as a cord wrapped tightly around the neck of the infant in a breech position.

When the weight of each mother, taken 3 months after delivery, was compared with her weight prior to pregnancy, it was found that the average gain for the entire group was exactly 2 pounds. Dr. King points out that, according to insurance statistics, the average gain per year for unmarried women between the ages of 20 and 30 years—the ages when most women are having their babies—is 1 pound. Other statistics show that married women, even though they have no children, gain on the average an extra 1.2 pounds per year. In his study, therefore, the women gained slightly less than they would have been expected to gain if they had not been pregnant.

A few of Dr. King's patients gained excessively. He believes the reason a pregnant woman may overeat is psychological; she is driven to continuous eating by nervous tension brought on by worries. Perhaps she is distressed about her appearance, her restricted social activities, or a fear that her husband will not continue to love her. Dr. King finds that excess pounds are quickly lost as soon as she has her baby, sees that her husband still loves her, realizes that restricted activities have marvelous compensations, and is busy caring for her child.

No one is arguing for a gain of fat during a pregnancy unless a woman has been severely underweight before she became pregnant. The fact remains that hundreds of women lose 20 to 25 pounds at the time of their deliveries. The combined weight of the infant, the extra weight of an enlarged uterus, the amniotic lining to the uterus, the placenta, the quarts of amniotic fluid in which the baby grows, and the increased weight of the enlarged mammary glands may add up to 20 pounds or more. When the total gain is restricted to 16 pounds, as it is by some obstetricians, the calorie intake must be so low that in my opinion there are many actual dangers: toxemia; difficult delivery; an infant in poor physical condition; complications setting in after delivery; and failure to produce sufficient milk for the baby. All of these conditions result from malnutrition brought about because health-building foods contain calories as well as nutrients.

A good rule to follow is to forgo any food which cannot build health. When a food offers nutrients needed by you or your unborn infant, eat it and cut down calories in other foods or else let the weight gain be what it may. It is far better to reduce a few pounds after your delivery than to risk the penalties of malnutrition. Plenty of exercise is involved in caring for a baby and in getting up once or twice during a night to feed him. Pounds usually roll off at such a time whether you want them to or not.

Expected weight gains. Most obstetricians allow a gain of 18 to 20 pounds during your entire pregnancy. *This gain should be figured from your ideal weight.* If you weighed 110 pounds when you became pregnant though your ideal weight was 120 pounds, your weight at the end of pregnancy should be approximately 140 pounds (120 pounds ideal weight plus 20 pounds gain). On the other hand, if your ideal weight is 130 and you weighed 150 pounds when you became pregnant, you should gain little if any. If you weigh 150 pounds at the end of pregnancy, you will actually have reduced fat weight at the rate of about 2 pounds per month.

A study of a large group of pregnant women whose average total gain was 20 pounds showed that the average gain in pounds per month was as follows:

First three months	none
Fourth month	4
Fifth month	5
Sixth month	4
Seventh month	3
Eighth month	2
Ninth month	2
	—
Total gain	20

The fact that as a group there was no gain during the first 3 months probably means that though some women gained, others were so nauseated that they lost weight, thereby decreasing the average of the group. The greater gains during the fourth, fifth, and sixth months are caused chiefly by the enlargement of the uterus, the increasing size of the placenta and the amniotic lining, and the accumulation of fluid inside the uterus. Such factors are largely stabilized by the end of the seventh month, and further gains are mainly those of the increasing weight of the infant.

It is important for the expectant mother to understand at what rate she may gain. I frequently find women who, on discovering they have gained 5 pounds during the fifth month, visualize themselves as gaining 20 pounds more; they become panicky and forgo nutritious foods in an attempt to control their weight. Aside from the harm they may do to themselves and the baby, they usually become starved, then overeat, and perhaps gain more than they would have otherwise.

Proteins stick to your ribs. Dr. Holmes (ref. 3, p. 48) found that women eating 110 to 120 grams of protein daily gained an average of 18 pounds during pregnancy compared with an average gain of 26 pounds for women eating 60 to 70 grams of protein daily. Aside from the fact that you need a generous amount of protein at this time, proteins stick to your ribs and keep you from being hungry. If you must actually reduce, however, all proteins should be as free from fat as possible.

Select lean meats and broil, pan broil, or roast them. The only exception is liver, which can be sautéed in just enough fat to prevent it from sticking to the pan. Pork, which contains a large amount of fat ("lean" ham is 40 per cent fat), and fish canned in oil, such as tuna and sardines, should be avoided. The fat from canned tuna, however, can be drained or even washed off. Luncheon meats which appear greasy when allowed to stand in a warm room should be forgone; liverwurst, for example, averages 50 per cent fat. Other meats, fish, or fowl should be eaten in generous amounts, even twice daily if you desire. On the other hand, do not avoid fat completely. When no fat is eaten, foods leave the stomach so quickly that you are soon starved and may overeat or eat foods which cannot build health.

Eggs should be boiled or poached; if scrambled or made into an omelet, they should be cooked in skim milk rather than in fat. Buy the cheapest cheese you can find; the cheaper it is, the less fat it contains. Either continue to add ½ cup of powdered skim milk to 1 quart of fresh milk or increase your intake of fresh skim milk to 2 quarts daily; if you find that you are hungry, the 2 quarts of liquid will fill you up more. Since brewers' yeast is 46 to 50 per cent protein and contains almost no fat and little digestible carbohydrate, use yeast as a dependable source of B vitamins rather than wheat germ, which is higher in calories. If wheat germ is avoided, however, be absolutely sure to obtain vitamin E daily in capsule form. In case you want to keep your calories to a minimum, the yeast can be stirred into water instead of fruit juice, but it is far less palatable. If you drink the yeast about ½ hour before meals, it will take the edge off your appetite.

Most fruits contain a generous quantity of natural sugar; eat them only in moderate amounts, especially if canned or cooked and sweetened. Instead of drinking orange juice, which leaves the stomach quickly, you will feel less hungry if you eat whole oranges. Dried fruits (which contain 75 per cent sugar), fresh persimmons (30 per cent sugar), and avocados (26 per cent fat) had better be avoided.

Vegetables supply approximately the same vitamins and minerals as do fruits; yet they contain far less sugar. The fresh vegetables which grow above the ground supply fewer calories than do roots or tubers. Raw vegetables, because of their harder texture, digest much less completely and hence supply fewer calories than do cooked vegetables. For example, it has been found that 38 calories are obtained from 1 ounce of cooked potato compared with only 18 calories from the same amount of raw potato. One of the easiest ways to maintain your weight or to reduce, therefore, is to become a raw-vegetable addict.

Have salads twice daily but keep largely to finger salads which call for no dressing: celery and carrot sticks; sliced tomatoes and cucumbers; green onions and radishes; or mounds of watercress and other greens. If you use French dressing or mayonnaise, restrict the amount to 1 teaspoon per salad. Boiled dressing is permitted or a dressing of yogurt, seasoned with catsup, Worcestershire, herbs, or whatever you desire. Avoid any dressing which contains mineral oil.

Limit yourself daily to one or two slices of bread, which should be 100 per cent whole wheat. Butter, cream, salad oils, and other fats should be used only in small quantities, and sugar, honey, jam, jellies, pastries, cookies, pie, cake, desserts, soft drinks, and alcoholic beverages should be avoided. If you feel you must go on a carbohydrate binge, eat angel food cake instead of candy or cookies; at least you will get some protein from the cake.

Your basic meal pattern may be somewhat as follows:

BREAKFAST:

    calcium tablets and/or iron or mixed-mineral tablets
    1 vitamin-C tablet, 100 milligrams, if no citrus fruit is to be eaten
    1 heaping tablespoon yeast taken in 8 ounces water or 4 ounces each water and juice
    1 sliced orange, ½ grapefruit, 1 peach, 2 apricots or plums, or small serving melon or unsweetened berries
    1 egg poached, boiled, or scrambled in skim milk
    1 glass skim milk
    1 slice whole-wheat toast with 1 teaspoon butter

1 cup coffee, black, no sugar (saccharine and milk if desired)
1 vitamin-A capsule, 25,000 units
1 vitamin-E capsule, 30 milligrams
1 vitamin-D capsule, 25,000 units taken every Sunday unless 2,000
   units are obtained daily with vitamin A

MIDMORNING:

1 glass skim milk

BEFORE LUNCH:

1 heaping tablespoon yeast in 8 ounces water or in 4 ounces each
   water and juice

LUNCH:

calcium tablets and/or iron or mixed-mineral tablets
1 vitamin-C tablet, 100 milligrams
lean meat (preferably liver) or fish or fowl; or egg if none for breakfast; or cheese or cream soup made of skim milk fortified with
   powdered skim milk
finger salad
2 glasses skim milk or 1 glass fortified milk

MIDAFTERNOON:

1 glass skim milk
1 orange or fresh peach or 2 plums or apricots

BEFORE DINNER:

1 heaping tablespoon yeast in 8 ounces water or in 4 ounces each
   water and juice

DINNER:

calcium tablets and/or iron or mixed-mineral tablets
vitamin-C tablet, 100 milligrams
fish, fruit, or tomato juice cocktail or bouillon if desired
meat, fish, or fowl
1 cooked vegetable
finger salad or salad with boiled dressing or yogurt or 1 teaspoon
   French dressing or mayonnaise
2 glasses skim milk or 1 glass fortified milk
no dessert or raw, unsweetened fruit

BEFORE BED:

1 glass skim milk

calcium and/or iron or mixed-mineral tablets and 1 vitamin-C
tablet if missed during the day

Let us now select specific menus and see if the calories are
behaving themselves:

Food	Calories	Alternatives
BREAKFAST		
vitamin-C and calcium or mineral tablets	0	
1 heaping tablespoon yeast in water	80	
in 4 ounces each pineapple juice * and water		67
1 sliced orange, medium	56	
1 egg, poached	75	
1 strip bacon, lean and well drained	56	
1 glass skim milk	84	
1 slice whole-wheat toast	75	
1 teaspoon butter on toast	33	
1 cup coffee, black, no sugar	0	
1 vitamin-A capsule	4	
1 vitamin-E capsule	4	
MIDMORNING:		
1 glass skim milk	84	
BEFORE LUNCH:		
1 heaping tablespoon yeast in water	80	
in 4 ounces each canned grapefruit juice * and water		50
LUNCH:		
vitamin-C and calcium or mineral tablets	0	
½ cup cottage cheese	90	
finger salad of cucumber, 14 slices	14	
2 carrots cut into sticks	15	
2 stalks celery	14	
1 medium tomato sliced or sectioned	32	
2 glasses skim milk	168	
MIDAFTERNOON:		
1 orange, medium	56	
1 glass skim milk	84	

Food	Calories	Alternatives
BEFORE DINNER:		
1 heaping tablespoon yeast in water	80	
in 4 ounces each water and apple juice *		59
DINNER:		
vitamin-C and calcium or mineral tablets	0	
shrimp cocktail	20	
liver, sautéed, generous serving	125	
½ cup string beans	28	
tossed salad	25	
with 1 teaspoon oil in dressing	33	
2 glasses skim milk	168	
1 medium fresh peach	45	
BEFORE BED:		
1 glass skim milk	84	
Total for entire day	1,712	1,888

* Different juices are given to show relative caloric values.

Since the usual caloric allowance is 2,500 calories per day during the last half of pregnancy, and since there are 4,000 calories in a pound of fat, if you stayed on a diet similar to the one outlined (leaving a deficit of 600 to 800 calories daily), you would lose about 1 pound of fat every 5 days or at least each week. Fortunately most women do not need to watch their weight so closely. Usually they can eat more bread, butter, cereals, cheeses, and other nutritious foods not suggested on the reducing diet.

Health comes first. Most persons planning to reduce start with a copious amount of good intentions, but their enthusiasm wanes as difficulties are encountered. Regardless of how much you need to reduce, always keep uppermost in your mind that your own welfare and that of your unborn infant come first. For example, you may decide to eat oranges instead of drinking the juice, but find that you do not get time to eat them or have failed to eat them because you went shopping or because it was just too much trouble. If this is the case, drink orange juice. Maybe you decide to cut calories by mixing yeast in water only to find it so unpalatable that you do not drink it; then by all means drink it in your favorite juice. If drinking 2 quarts of milk daily makes you so full that you are miserable, beat ½ cup of powdered milk into 1 quart of fresh milk and drink the smaller amount every day. If you are still too full to be comfortable, make tigers' milk (p. 31) and eliminate the liquid you would otherwise drink with yeast. In other words, make your diet practical for yourself.

Although it is possible to stay on a diet quite restricted as to calories and yet obtain the nutrients necessary to meet the requirements of pregnancy, it is not easy. One obstetrician tells me that he gives this advice to his patients: "Watch your calories on everything else, but if a food contains protein, the more you eat of it, the better." Not a bad bit of advice.

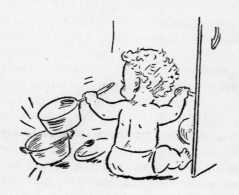

CHAPTER 7

ADVANTAGES OF NURSING
AND REASONS FOR FAILURES

IT IS conceded that breast milk is the ideal food for infants. In the past, mothers eager to nurse their babies have frequently been discouraged from doing so by nurses and pediatricians who have encountered difficulties with breast feeding. This attitude is gradually changing, however, since it is now recognized that psychological rewards are to be gained by both mother and baby through nursing. Many a young mother may still meet opposition in her desire to nurse her infant. She could argue, as could anyone, the relative advantages of nursing versus bottle feeding for endless hours; yet each arguer would probably keep his own convictions on the subject.

Suffice it to say that if you wish to nurse your baby, *do not let anyone or anything discourage you.* If your desire is strong enough, the chances are that you will succeed. There are degrees, however, of wanting to nurse your baby. One mother will give up at the least discouragement, whereas another will fight to the last tooth and nail.

Breast-fed babies have higher resistance to infections. Dr. Naish,[1] a practicing pediatrician, investigated a series of infants suffering with enteritis, or inflammation of the intestine. Somewhat to her surprise, she found that almost 75 per cent of the babies who had been breast fed for a month or longer recovered from the illness, whereas more than 70 per cent of the infants

---

[1] F. C. Naish, "Morbidity and Feeding in Infancy," *Lancet,* 1 (1949), 146.

who had never been breast fed failed to recover. She points out that one reason she and her fellow pediatricians are not more insistent upon breast feeding is that they see too few breast-fed babies to be continually reminded of how superior these babies are to bottle-fed ones; that mothers often do not take breast-fed babies to a physician because they are so healthy; and the babies are so infrequently ill that doctors are rarely called into the homes to see them. In going over her own records of infants who had suffered from infections, she found that for every home call she had made to see an ill breast-fed baby, she had made four calls to see babies who had been only partially breast fed and six calls to see babies who had never been breast fed.

Numerous other studies have shown that breast-fed babies have higher resistance to infections than do bottle-fed ones. The classic of these studies was made by Dr. Grulee [2] when professor of pediatrics at the University of Illinois School of Medicine. He and his associates, working through the Infant Welfare Society in Chicago, followed all babies under 1 year until the total had reached 20,000 infants. They found that the bottle-fed babies suffered twice as many infections as did the breast-fed infants and that ten times more of them died from infections. Of all the babies suffering from infections, 66.1 per cent had been completely bottle fed, 27.2 per cent had been partially breast fed, and only 6.7 per cent wholly breast fed. Of the infants who died of respiratory infections, 96.7 per cent had been wholly or partially bottle fed and only 3.3 per cent completely breast fed. It was also found that bottle-fed infants suffered three times more gastrointestinal infections than did the breast-fed babies. Dr. Grulee and his coworkers conclude that "breast feeding gives a much greater immunity to infections than does artificial feeding," and that "even partial breast feeding gives considerable immunity."

[2] C. G. Grulee, H. N. Sanford, and P. H. Herron, "Breast and Artificial Feeding; Influence on Morbidity and Mortality on Twenty Thousand Infants," *Journal of the American Medical Association,* 103 (1934), 735.

Dr. Ebbs,[3] professor of pediatrics at the University of Toronto College of Medicine, found almost the same immunity among breast-fed babies in his study of 1,500 sick infants. Four times as many of the bottle-fed infants suffered from acute infections as did the breast-fed babies. When infants had been breast fed until they were 6 weeks old, only half as many suffered from infections as did infants wholly bottle fed. A large number of bottle-fed babies died from infections, whereas most of the breast-fed babies recovered. When the dead infants were autopsied, it was found that almost every baby who had been bottle fed had suffered from sinusitis and from infections in the middle ear.

Such statistics would be depressing for a mother to contemplate if she had to watch her pitifully sick infant, perhaps her only child, fight for air, especially when she remembers that she made little or no attempt to nurse him. These statistics are cruel to a heartbroken mother who sits helplessly by and sees her baby die, realizing that she might have prevented that death if she had tried harder. Yet statistics are cold, meaningless things until your own baby becomes a statistic with an entry on a hospital chart which perhaps says, "Died at 2:03 A.M. Acute bronchitis." After that you can never forget their meaning. If you make no attempt to nurse your baby, you may tell yourself that he will stay well. I hope you are right, but hundreds of mothers who are no longer mothers also believed that.

How immunity is produced. Although the means by which immunity is produced through breast feeding is not entirely understood, it is known that breast milk contains antibodies capable of fighting numerous infections and that antibodies to human diseases are not found in cows' milk. Whenever a mother has suffered from an infection or has been exposed to an infection, her liver produces antibodies which from that time on circulate in her blood. Breast milk, formed as her blood circulates through the mammary glands, will contain antibodies in proportion to the

[3] J. H. Ebbs and F. Mulligan, "The Incidence of Mortality of Breast and Artificially Fed Infants Admitted to the Hospital with Infections," *Arch. Dis. Childhood*, **17** (1942), 217.

number and kind in her blood serum. If a baby is so fortunate as to be nursed through most of his first year, he is continuously supplied with antibodies which he himself has no possibility of producing unless he is first exposed to each specific type of disease-producing bacteria.

It has also been found that artificially fed babies suffer ten times more frequently from allergies than do breast-fed infants. Some evidence indicates that when a foreign material, or antigen, capable of causing an allergy, gets into the blood of a healthy individual, antibodies are sometimes produced which render the antigen harmless. These protective substances may be secreted in a mother's milk and guard her infant from attack by similar antigens. The relation of breast feeding to infrequent allergies, however, may be only because breast-fed babies are cuddled, rocked, and held during feedings more often than are artificially fed ones.

Sore breasts and cracked nipples. Thousands of women have wanted to nurse their infants, but sore breasts have resulted in such excruciating pain that nursing became impossible. As was shown by the Harvard and Toronto studies, when the prenatal diets have been adequate, the incidence of inflammation, infections, and abscesses of the breast is markedly decreased. If the mother is sufficiently aware of nutrition to attempt to produce breast milk of the highest quality (p. 81), the amount of protein and of vitamins A, C, and E will help to protect her mammary glands from bacterial invasion.

The fact remains, however, that breast milk, like any other form of milk, is an ideal food in which bacteria can multiply with breath-taking speed. Since bacteria are ever present and the nipple holes are open, any milk oozing from the breast or dried around the nipples fosters the growth of billions of bacteria, which can readily pass into the mammary glands. The reason a mother is advised to sponge her breasts thoroughly before and especially after each nursing is not to protect her infant from bacteria half so much as to protect herself from infection and the excruciating pain which may result.

So-called caked breast is actually an infection in the mammary glands which causes them to be so swollen that the entire breast appears to be caked. The home remedy for caked breast a half century ago was to keep the entire breast covered with piping-hot pancakes, an interesting substitute for our modern heating pads. In addition to whatever treatment your physician recommends, you should see that your protein intake is unusually high, increase vitamin A to 50,000 units after each meal, and obtain 100 milligrams of vitamin C every 2 or 3 hours until the infection subsides.

Cracked nipples usually occur when the diet has been deficient in protein or vitamin C or when the nipples have not been toughened by sufficient brushing or manipulation before the baby was born. As a rule the condition is readily healed when protein and vitamin C are generously supplied. Recently a young mother phoned to ask if she should let her infant nurse when the milk contained so much blood from her cracked nipples that it was discolored. I explained to her that many people considered the drinking of blood to be particularly health building and bought it from a slaughterhouse for that reason. In addition to checking her protein intake, I suggested that she take 100 milligrams of vitamin C every 2 hours for 3 days. Her nipples healed rapidly, and she continued to nurse her baby without further difficulty.

Other reasons for nursing failures. Physicians grant that your ability to nurse your baby will depend upon your desire to do so and the frequency of putting the baby to the breast. They also stress, however, that milk production is limited by heredity, your endocrine balance, and the development of your mammary glands and nipples. These arguments may be perfectly true but sound formidable if any difficulty arises. Certainly you cannot grow new breasts or nipples, change your heredity, or obtain other sets of glands. Nevertheless the fact remains that throughout the thousands of decades of human existence and up until the past 50 years, practically 100 per cent of billions of mothers have nursed their babies. It is doubtful that there has been much change in heredity, the endocrine glands, or the structure of breasts in the past half century.

What has changed is that the diets have become progressively more deficient as a greater number of refined foods have become available and inexpensive. Furthermore, babies were formerly born at home, put to the breast almost immediately, and allowed to nurse thereafter every time they wished; during the past few decades most babies have been born in hospitals where the mother may not see her infant for a day or two and then for only a few fleeting moments.

Hospital routines and the belief that a baby should be kept on a 4-hour schedule have been largely responsible for failures in cases where mothers wished to nurse their infants. When a baby is brought to his mother for only 15 minutes every 4 hours during the day and not at all during the night, there is not time for sufficient sucking to stimulate milk flow. If no supplementary food has been given, a strong infant may be starved after a 4-hour wait; he may tear into the breast like a young wolf, causing the nipples to become so sore that nursing may have to be stopped. Gentle sucking at frequent intervals rarely causes the breasts to be painful. Furthermore, pediatricians, as a matter of pride, want babies to regain their birth weight as quickly as possible; for this reason they often order formulas to be given in the hospital nursery; a baby who is not really hungry when brought to his mother will nurse too little to stimulate the milk flow. Dr. Grulee of Chicago was able to increase the number of nursing mothers under his care from 50 to 90 per cent merely by not allowing any baby to have a supplementary feeding during the first week.

Sucking stimulates milk flow. Numerous studies have been made of the effect of sucking on stimulating milk flow. The results boil down to one sentence: the more frequently the infant sucks at first, or until a normal milk flow is established, the greater the supply of milk, particularly if the baby nurses both breasts at each feeding. When infants are allowed to nurse as frequently as they wish, the number of times some babies will nurse is truly astonishing. A baby in a Detroit hospital where infants were kept with the mothers nursed twenty-three times during a single day. Most mothers react to such information by exclaiming, "Heavens! How could I ever get my housework done?" The points to remember are that the more the infant nurses at first, the sooner the milk flow is established, the more quickly the baby will get sufficient milk at each feeding, and the earlier he will put himself on a 3- or 4-hour schedule.

The importance of sucking in stimulating milk flow is shown by the experience of a friend of mine, the mother of five boys. She had wanted desperately to nurse her first three babies, but the usual hospital routine and the belief that a 4-hour schedule must be maintained had entirely defeated her. Before the birth of her fourth child, however, she read articles in popular magazines about the importance of sucking and of allowing an infant to select his own feeding schedule. She was determined to try again. Since babies were not allowed to stay in their mothers' rooms, she left the hospital when her baby was less than 48 hours old so that he could nurse as much as he wished. She had arranged for her young sister to stay with the other children and to run the house. According to the sister the infant "nursed all day long." In any case he nursed so much that the sister would frequently exclaim, "What? Nursing him again! You can have it. I'll take office work." This mother tells me that her breasts were tender but not sore, and that in 2 or 3 days she had more milk than the baby could take. Afterward he nursed every 3 or 4 hours. She is now nursing her fifth boy with no trouble whatsoever.

Fortunately almost every city has or will soon have at least one hospital where a baby can "room in" with his mother. If you are sure at the beginning of your pregnancy that you want to nurse your baby, you should select your obstetrician from among those who take their cases to such a hospital. I know of a number of mothers who have worked backward in determining which obstetrician to go to. They called the hospitals in their city until they found one or more which allow "rooming in"; they learned from the hospital office which obstetricians deliver babies at that hospital; then they made their selection accordingly. A morning thus spent at the telephone can bring rich rewards.

Milk flow can be stimulated later. It is usually assumed that if the milk flow is not adequate when the baby is 2 or 3 weeks old, there is nothing to do except to give a supplement. The quantity of breast milk can usually be increased at any time if the mother will make the effort to cause it to increase. Supplementary feedings should, of course, be given whenever they are needed, but if the mother wishes to continue nursing, her first thought should be to stimulate the milk flow.

Twice I have run across articles in the medical literature which are so unusual that I hesitate to quote them. One report was of Mundugumor women [4] in New Guinea who, although they had never been pregnant, often adopt young infants, and by putting them to the breast and allowing them to suck all they wished, were able to secrete enough milk to feed them. The other report told of peasant women in Sicily who were able to nurse infants even though they themselves had not been pregnant.

Simarian and Miau [4] give the case history of a woman whose success at nursing they considered to be outstanding. This mother had been delivered by Caesarean section and had stayed in the hospital for 16 days. Her infant had not been put to the breast, and the amount of her milk had been negligible. The first day she was home, when the baby was 16 days old, she allowed him to nurse as much as he would, weighing him before and after each nursing. Since he obtained only 3.5 ounces of milk, a supplement was given. During the following week the baby nursed fifty-two times. The milk flow gradually increased, and by the time he was 22 days old, he was obtaining 17.5 ounces of milk. No more supplements were used after that time.

A far more spectacular case was told to me by Mrs. Gladys Lindberg, a nutrition consultant. A young woman came to her with a baby 6 weeks old. Although the mother had had plenty of milk, her nipples were so badly inverted that the hospital physician had told her it would be impossible for the baby to nurse; hence he had never been put to the breast. The infant had not thrived. His formula had been changed several times;

[4] F. P. Simarian and F. Miau, "Breast Feeding," *Journal of Pediatrics,* 33 (1948), 295.

yet he was a weak, whimpering little thing who continued to lose weight. The mother was penniless and desperate.

Mrs. Lindberg advised the mother to put the baby to the breast and allow him to suck as much as he would. When he would no longer suck either breast without crying, she was to give him just enough formula to satisfy his most severe hunger pains, thus making sure he would want to nurse soon again. Her inverted nipples, gently massaged, became sufficiently firm and protruding for the baby to nurse. Mrs. Lindberg outlined a diet for the woman to follow, supplying her with powdered milk, yeast, and wheat germ. The infant started to thrive immediately, and within a few days the formula was discontinued. The mother nursed the child completely for a full year.

The most interesting part of this case we discovered only after I had asked Mrs. Lindberg to check every detail for accuracy before I wrote about it. On going to the mother's home, Mrs. Lindberg found that the baby, now a beautiful boy of 2, was the picture of health. Money is still scarce, however, and the mother has not been able to buy as much milk as she would like her son to have. She is, therefore, still nursing him each night as she rocks him to drowsiness. Shocking? Perhaps to persons who have never known poverty. A mother who will do that for her child has my wholehearted admiration, and I imagine she has yours too.

Dr. Margaret Mead, the famous anthropologist, who has studied primitive races throughout the world, says that she has never heard of a native woman unable to nurse her baby; that foster mothers suckle infants only when the natural mother is already nursing one or more other babies or has died. There are cases on record of primitive women suckling as many as five children at one time. A pediatrician who worked at the Chicago Lying-in Hospital told me that several of their wet nurses sold 80 and 90 ounces of milk daily for years after a pregnancy. In all probability, nature intended every woman's breasts to be functional.

CHAPTER 8

STIMULATING BREAST MILK

I F YOUR flow of milk has been established, success or failure in nursing your baby from then on is largely determined by the adequacy or inadequacy of your diet.

From the point of view of nutrition the principal reason for the increasing numbers of nursing failures is that the consumption of foods rich in proteins and B vitamins has steadily decreased. Dr. Norman Jolliffe, professor at Cornell University Medical School, estimated that persons in poorhouses a century ago obtained some five times more B vitamins than even well-to-do people do today. Until the past few decades, protein foods were abundant and inexpensive and formed a principal part of the diet because few fruits and vegetables were available.

Factors which increase the quantity of milk. An adequate diet for a nursing mother is essentially the same as that needed during the last months of pregnancy (p. 35). The need for calcium, protein, and especially the B vitamins, however, has increased. Research with experimental animals has shown that the requirement of B vitamins during lactation sometimes increases as much as five times or more over the usual amount needed. To obtain such a quantity becomes an almost superhuman feat considering that it is difficult to meet even minimum requirements from our average American diet.

Dr. Icie Macy, working with the Children's Fund of Michigan, is undoubtedly the world's authority on any detail pertaining to breast milk. Her findings show that the eating of foods rich in carbohydrates (starches and sugars) increases the fat content of milk but does not increase the flow. Eating foods high in fat also increases the richness of breast milk and increases the flow slightly. The quantity of breast milk, however, has been found to be increased in proportion to the amount of protein eaten and the quantity of B vitamins obtained. If the diet consists largely of foods rich in protein and the B vitamins, the output of milk is then limited only by such factors as heredity, mammary-gland development, and endocrine balance.

Contrary to popular opinion, the drinking of excessive amounts of liquids such as water, tea, coffee, and soft drinks does not increase the quantity of milk. The nursing mother's liquid intake, of course, should be adequate and has been estimated to be between 2 and 3 quarts daily. The drinking of fresh milk stimulates the flow of breast milk largely because of the protein and vitamin B_2, or riboflavin, it supplies.

Some time ago certain vitamins were found to stimulate milk flow so remarkably that they were called L_1 and L_2, or lactation vitamins. It now appears that these substances are one and the same thing: the B vitamin, inositol, which is particularly rich in blackstrap molasses. It is also found in yeast, liver, wheat germ, and whole-grain breads and cereals.

The old wives' tale that beer stimulated the production of breast milk was scientifically sound as long as brewers' yeast was left in the beer. Such beer supplied three needs of the mother: the B vitamins, protein, and liquid. Imported beer coming from Denmark or Sweden probably has 2 tablespoons or more of yeast in each pint bottle. The yeast has been removed from American beers; hence the B vitamins and protein are lacking.

Since dry brewers' yeast is 46 per cent protein or more, contains all the known B vitamins, and is customarily taken in liquid, it becomes the modern substitute for old-fashioned beer. I have made out lactation diets for hundreds of women, and it has been my experience that if a mother will take as much as 3 heaping tablespoons of yeast every day, she will have enough milk for her baby. As soon as she gives up the yeast, her milk flow decreases or ceases.

A few years ago, a young woman who had come to me for advice throughout her pregnancy had so much breast milk that she sold the excess to a hospital. Though she hated the taste of yeast, she needed the money the hospital paid her. Time and again she would fail to take yeast, and on the following day she would have no milk to sell. When she took as much as 3 heaping tablespoons of yeast daily, she was able to sell 30 ounces (or more) of breast milk over that which her own baby could drink.

The relation of the mother's diet to the quality of breast milk. The quality of breast milk depends almost directly upon the adequacy of the mother's diet. With the exception of calcium and phosphorus, if nutrients are not supplied in the mother's diet, they cannot be secreted in the milk.

When the mother fails to obtain enough calcium and phosphorus to meet her own needs and those of the breast milk, these minerals are withdrawn from her bones and teeth and passed on to her infant. Dozens of studies have shown that the nursing mother is usually in what is spoken of as negative calcium balance. That is, more calcium is excreted in her breast milk and in her urine and feces than is supplied by her diet. On the other hand, if the mother takes sufficient calcium in the form of both milk and mineral tablets, no minerals are withdrawn from her teeth and bones, and the amount of calcium in the breast milk can be slightly increased. It is, therefore, more important to take calcium tablets while you are nursing your baby than during pregnancy.

If a mother's diet is somewhat inadequate in protein, the quantity of breast milk is decreased. If her diet becomes still more deficient in protein, the production of breast milk further decreases or ceases.

Only the vitamins of the B group appear to affect the quantity of breast milk produced. The amount of vitamins A, C, D, E, and perhaps K secreted in the milk, however, is in proportion to the quantity supplied by the mother's diet. It has been found that the vitamin-A content of breast milk can be considerably increased if the mother takes daily as much as 50,000 units of the vitamin or more. The minimum vitamin-C requirements of the infant can be met if the mother obtains 150 milligrams of the vitamin daily, but she must take 300 milligrams or more before the milk contains enough of this vitamin to keep the infant's tissues saturated, a condition considered to be ideal. An infant's minimum need for vitamin D apparently can be supplied in breast milk provided the mother obtains 2,000 units or more daily; no vitamin D whatsoever is found in breast milk when the mother herself lacks this nutrient. In contrast with cows' milk which contains little or none of vitamins E and K, breast milk can be a rich source of both. The mother, however, must obtain enough of these vitamins in her own diet or have favorable bacteria growing in her intestines which can synthesize vitamin K. Some breast milk supplies no vitamin K, but if the mother eats cabbage (preferably as cole slaw), or spinach, the two richest sources, her milk furnishes both vitamins.

The average breast milk contains too few B vitamins to meet the optimum requirements of a baby. In this respect the mother's needs have priority over those of her infant. Dr. Macy found, however, that if the nursing mother would eat liver daily, the amount of B vitamins, particularly of biotin, inositol, and pantothenic acid, in her milk could be markedly increased.

The value of the first milk produced. The milk secreted by the mother during the first 5 days of her infant's life is spoken of as colostrum. It would appear that nature designed colostrum to give the infant a good start, so rich is it in certain nutrients. For example, later breast milk averages 1.06 per cent protein,[1] whereas colostrum has been found to be as high as 6.8 per cent. The vitamin-A content of colostrum averages five times that of later breast milk, and the carotene content averages twelve times that of later milk. Since infants store little or no vitamin A before birth, the high vitamin-A and carotene content of colostrum is particularly valuable to them. It has also been found that antibodies and antitoxins [2] are sometimes three or four times more

---

[1] Icie G. Macy, "Composition of Human Colostrum and Mature Breast Milk," *American Journal of the Diseases of Children,* **78** (1949), 589.

[2] J. Liebling and H. E. Schmitz, "Colostrum as a Source of Diphtheria Antitoxin," *J. Pediat.,* **22** (1943), 189.

concentrated in colostrum than in the breast milk secreted later. It is well to remember that infants are particularly susceptible to such infections as bronchitis and pneumonia, and many of them die during their first month of life from these diseases. How often have such infants been kept in hospital nurseries and not allowed to have their mothers' colostrum?

If you do not wish to nurse your baby at any other time, be humane enough to nurse him during his first 5 days of life.

A milk-producing diet. To supply sufficient milk for your baby is not enough. If he is to grow normally and to remain healthy, your milk must also be of high quality.

There are a few general rules to follow. Put the foods rich in proteins and B vitamins on the "must" list: liver, wheat germ, and yeast. Eat one or more of these foods daily, the more the better. Have 1 quart of skim milk daily, and preferably 1½ quarts; fortify every drop of milk you drink by beating ½ cup of powdered skim milk into it (p. 25). See that you use approximately 3 quarts of liquid daily. Because of the inositol content of blackstrap molasses, take 1 tablespoon or more every day. These items alone should take care of quantity. To assure breast milk of high quality and to protect yourself, obtain ample amounts of all known nutrients.

Your daily schedule may be somewhat as follows:

BREAKFAST:
2 calcium tablets or tablets of mixed minerals
1 glass (8 ounces) freshly squeezed orange juice
wheat germ as a cereal or with a cooked or cold cereal, toasted if desired
1 egg and/or bacon if desired
toasted whole-wheat or wheat-germ bread
1 glass fortified milk or tigers' milk (p. 31)
coffee if desired, preferably black; no more than 1 cup
1 or 2 vitamin-A capsules, 25,000 units each
vitamin-D capsule at least 2,000 units, if taken daily
vitamin-E capsule, 30 milligrams, unless ½ cup of wheat germ has been eaten

1 tablespoon blackstrap molasses, taken directly from a spoon unless used in tigers' milk

MIDMORNING:

1 heaping tablespoon yeast in juice or in tigers' milk
cheese and crackers if desired

LUNCH:

2 calcium tablets or tablets of mixed minerals
1 vitamin-C tablet, 100 milligrams
meat, preferably liver or liverwurst, or eggs or cottage cheese or a milk soup fortified with powdered milk
fruit or vegetable or salad of either
fortified milk, preferably 2 glasses, or 1 glass tigers' milk
fruit or milk dessert if desired

MIDAFTERNOON:

1 heaping tablespoon yeast in juice or in tigers' milk
small peanut-butter sandwich made with wheat-germ or whole-wheat bread

DINNER:

2 calcium tablets or tablets of mixed minerals
1 vitamin-C tablet, 100 milligrams
meat (preferably liver if none at lunch) or fish or fowl
1 or 2 cooked vegetables
salad, preferably with cottage cheese
fortified milk or tigers' milk
fruit or milk dessert if desired

BEFORE RETIRING:

1 heaping tablespoon of yeast in juice or tigers' milk
finish fortified milk if less than 1 quart has been drunk during the day

As in the preceding chapters, the position on the menu of the vitamin and mineral preparations indicates whether they should be taken before or after a meal.

How to tell when a baby is hungry. One of the problems in nursing a baby is the difficulty of determining whether or not the infant is getting enough to eat. If, after the baby has nursed, he screams until he is purple and pulls up his legs as if in pain, even an experienced mother may not know whether the child is still hungry, needs to be burped, or is suffering from colic. The hungry baby is in pain; his stomach hurts him. Dr. Brown,[3] professor of pediatrics at the University of Toronto Medical School, points out that for one nursing baby who gets too much milk, physicians see 99 babies who are still hungry after being nursed, especially following the evening feeding when the mother is tired and has less milk than at other times.

Dr. Brown stresses that a baby continually hungry is unusually alert and holds his head up better than do other babies, his back tensed; that he is a light sleeper; and that his mother is usually complimented by friends remarking that they have never seen such an intelligent-looking baby. This physician compares such a baby with a hungry puppy, the runt which is crowded out but soon becomes a favorite because in its search for food it is alert, wakeful, and full of pep. A full puppy, according to Dr. Brown, is lazy, stupid, and relaxed, and the full infant is similarly "a stupid little animal." (Shall we let Dr. Brown get away with that?) If a baby is wakeful, alert, and intelligent looking, and handles himself too well for his age, this doctor's advice is to give him a supplementary feeding whenever he cries after being nursed.

When a supplement must be given. Rather than the somewhat confusing terms of complementary and supplementary feedings, I merely use the term supplement to mean any bottle feeding given to a nursing baby. The starting of such feeding is usually the beginning of the end of nursing. Thousands of mothers have found supplementary feedings too difficult and understandably so. The technics used in the past and sometimes still in use are enough to discourage anyone.

I do not know of anything which seems to me to be so utterly ridiculous as weighing a baby before and after each nursing and

[3] A. Brown, "Scientific Construction of the Normal Child's Diet," *Lancet,* 2 (1948), 877.

then forcing enough formula on him to bring the total feeding to a certain number of ounces. It would make just as much sense to weigh a kitten before and after it laps up milk and then try to force it to drink more.

No two babies desire the same quantity of milk at each feeding, nor does one baby wish to eat the same amount at every feeding during the day. Allow the baby to take what breast milk you have and as much supplement as he wants, and let it go at that. If he dozes off to sleep without a supplement, so much the better provided you have time to allow him to nurse often; he will soon become hungry again, and by frequent nursing may stimulate milk flow until the supplement can be discontinued. If, after you have allowed him to nurse both breasts, he shows the alertness stressed by Dr. Brown, still cries, chews his fists, and revolves his head with lips pursed and mouth open every time a cheek is touched, you can be quite sure he would like something more to eat. In that case, let him take as much supplement as he wants. The only exception is when you are trying to increase your milk flow by having the baby suck as much as he will; at such a time let him have only enough formula to keep him temporarily happy.

Another accepted procedure which has made it difficult for mothers to give supplementary feedings is the mixing of complicated formulas and the sterilizing of mixing bowls, measuring cups, bottles and nipples, all without knowing whether or not the baby will take any of the food. The nursing itself is time-consuming; if the infant is young, at least 30 minutes will be required at each nursing for him to drain both breasts. It takes more time to sterilize the equipment and make and give a formula, in addition to breast feeding, than most mothers can give. The problem, therefore, is one of simplification.

Dr. McCulloch, professor of clinical pediatrics at Washington University Medical School, appears to have the answer. He recommends (ref. 3, p. 116) that no sugar of any kind be added to an infant's formula; that the formula be made merely of evaporated milk and water. I was at first amazed and then delighted to read of his advising his patients to give an infant water which has not been boiled provided the water is safe for an adult to drink, is added to the formula immediately before being given to the baby, and any remaining formula is thrown away. Evaporated milk, of course, is already sterile. As in the case of preparing orange juice for an infant, there is no need to sterilize the bottles and nipples; when the juice (or formula) is given immediately after being prepared, there is no time for bacteria to multiply. Thus the work is lessened in preparing supplements.

The procedure, therefore, is roughly this: let your baby nurse from both breasts as long as he will. If he still seems hungry, put a pacifier in his mouth to keep him from being fretful while you pour 1 or 2 ounces of evaporated milk directly into a clean (not necessarily sterilized) bottle, add an equal amount of warm water (from the tap if your tap water is safe for you to drink), cover the bottle with a clean (not necessarily sterilized) nipple, and give it to the baby. The whole procedure will take from 2 to 5 minutes. If you cannot give the infant more of your time, it is better to prop the bottle in a bottle holder than to discontinue nursing because of the time it takes.

The hardest part of this technic is getting accustomed to the idea yourself. The first time I gave our baby daughter a formula made with tap water without first sterilizing the bottle and nipple, I felt it would surely make her ill.

When the supply of breast milk is almost adequate, I frequently recommend that instead of giving a supplement, the mother give vegetable-cooking water (p. 134) to which is added a small amount of yeast. In many cases the procedure has worked out satisfactorily.

It seems to me there is too much of the all-or-none policy in changing from nursing to bottle feeding. When circumstances allow, why not continue nursing for one or two feedings during the day and give a formula at other times? Perhaps the best time to nurse the baby would be early in the morning when your breast milk is more plentiful and/or in the evening when you may most enjoy rocking him.

If you have enough milk to nurse your baby at all, the chances are that you can increase your milk supply so that you can nurse him entirely if you really wish to do so. A diet extremely high in protein and in all the B vitamins is necessary.

The over-the-hump diet. If it is possible to increase your supply of breast milk through nutrition, the increase will come within 3 days after you have started eating food known to stimulate milk production. Why not try to increase your milk supply? Let's call your food for these days the over-the-hump diet. After your milk production has increased, you can probably maintain it by following the diet outlined on page 83. For 3 days, however, try to eat the following amounts of each of these foods:

1 tablespoon blackstrap molasses, mixed with milk or taken directly from a spoon; 2 or 3 tablespoons if enjoyed

6 heaping tablespoons yeast, taken 1 before each meal, and/or 1 between meals, 1 before bed; take in tigers' milk or any juice you prefer

1 cup wheat germ; take ½ cup at breakfast and ½ cup for lunch or in the afternoon or before bed; toast it and eat it as a cold cereal

1 large serving of liver at lunch or dinner

1½ quarts skim milk with ½ cup powdered skim milk added to each quart; approximately 1 glass at each meal, 1 between meals, and 1 before bed

If you manage to eat these quantities, you will probably be too full to eat anything else; take your tablets or capsules and forget about other foods for the time being unless you want them. If you cannot eat these amounts, then do the best you can. I strongly suspect that this diet would make even a statue produce more milk than any baby could drink provided the food is digested and absorbed.

The effect of fatigue and loss of sleep. Probably every mother who has nursed a baby has found that her milk has been decreased by fatigue, worry, and loss of sleep. If her milk dries up, she usually believes it is because she worked too hard, became overtired, and probably lost sleep at the same time.

There is no doubt that rest and relaxation are tremendously

important. The direct cause of the decreased milk supply, how-ever, is probably not the lack of rest. The harder a person works or the more sleep he loses, the more his requirements of the B vitamins are increased; these vitamins are needed in proportion to the energy output. Since such large amounts of B vitamins are already needed for lactation, a slight deficiency quickly results both in fatigue and in the drying up of breast milk. When the diet is truly adequate, it is amazing how much physical work a mother can do without any decrease in her milk supply.

My friend with the five boys is a case in point. She does all of her own housework and keeps her home spotlessly clean. The amount of cooking, dish washing, laundering, ironing, and clean-ing she does is nothing less than staggering. Yet she somehow finds the energy to have fun with her boys, entertain guests, work in her garden, raise chickens, and do a hundred and one other things in addition to nursing her baby. How she keeps going on the amount of sleep she gets, I shall never know. She and I have what our husbands call the-coffee-and-baby club; every morning at a specified time each of us pours a cup of coffee and sits down to the phone to talk babies with one another. Almost daily she reports scrubbing kitchen walls or some such activity until well after midnight and then getting up at six in the morning. Yet her diet is excellent, and her breast milk remains adequate.

The young mother who sold breast milk is another example. She used to go out daily to clean homes and for a time cleaned for me. She would arrive early in the morning with her baby and sterile bottles; except for the time she spent nursing him and draining the remainder of her milk, she was scrubbing floors, washing windows, and doing every variety of difficult housework. She had plenty of milk for her own baby at all times and, as long as she took yeast, a surplus to sell.

One could cite hundreds of other examples of women who did physically strenuous work and still nursed their babies. Surely the pioneer wives who had many children and nursed them all did as much work as most mothers do today, if not more. It is doubtful that physical exertion can cause a decrease in breast milk as long as the diet is adequate.

Let your baby get acquainted with the bottle. Regardless of how abundant your milk supply may be, let your baby get acquainted with the bottle. Some unforeseen circumstance may arise which would make weaning necessary. Unless a baby has been offered a bottle from birth, he may refuse to drink from a rubber nipple, and a stormy session for both you and your infant may follow.

Dr. Lee Edward Travis, well known for his work in psychology, stresses that if a child is to grow up to be emotionally secure, he should be allowed to drink from a bottle until he is at least 2 years old. To prepare your baby for the time when you may wish to wean him, let him drink from a bottle daily throughout the nursing period. Perhaps your husband would be willing to give the baby a night or early morning formula while you sleep. If no supplementary feedings are desired, however, plain boiled water can be given. Orange juice, vegetable-cooking water, or the nutritional supplements suggested in the next chapter would be still better.

How long should nursing be continued? It seems to me that this question can be answered with one simple statement: as long as you and your baby both enjoy it. There is no set time. A week of nursing is better than none; 2 months is better than 1. The child who is nursed for 9 or 10 months is fortunate indeed. In many parts of the world children are nursed until they are 3 years old, and studies show that such children become emotionally stable and mentally sound adults, able to withstand far greater physical and psychological stress than we can endure.

I would say to nurse your baby as long as you want to; it is no one's business but your own. A number of mothers have told me that they cried the last time they nursed their babies. To meet such thoroughly feminine women is a joy, and one cannot help feeling that perhaps other mothers might be happier if they, too, felt like crying because they could no longer nurse their children.

Enjoy nursing your baby. A baby is tiny such a short time that it is a shame not to enjoy nursing him. Each new period of growth is fascinating, but the cuddly helplessness of the small baby, the warmth and intimacy between yourself and your infant, and the many charms of babyhood can never be recaptured. Relax and enjoy him while you can. Let your housework go if necessary; realize that only neurotics worry about what others may think of their housekeeping. Even if it stretches your budget to the limit, buy yourself a comfortable rocking chair. No matter how off key your voice, learn some lullabies. And know that nursing is something to be enjoyed rather than merely to be endured. The difference between enjoying nursing or not is largely one of attitude.

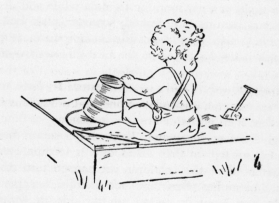

CHAPTER 9

ALL BABIES NEED
NUTRITIONAL SUPPLEMENTS

ALTHOUGH breast milk is undoubtedly the most nearly ideal food for an infant, it is not perfect. Nor is cows' milk perfect, since it is deficient in many essential nutrients. Before health can be produced, the nutrients lacking in milk should be added to the infant's diet.

The attitude of the Food and Drug Administration and of the Council of Foods and Nutrition of the American Medical Association toward many nutrients not yet proved to be necessary to human health is expressed by the statement, "The need in human nutrition has not been established." At the present writing, this attitude is taken toward such nutrients as several of the B vitamins, vitamins E and P, and certain unsaturated fatty acids. The above statement often misleads mothers and physicians alike into assuming that such nutrients are unimportant.

Although the need for vitamin K has only recently been established, it is now known that a lack of this vitamin can cause a baby's death. All of the nutrients not accepted as essential to human well-being have been used successfully in treating certain abnormalities in humans, and all are necessary to the health of experimental animals. As long as a nutrient is absolutely harmless and may be beneficial, it seems to me that it should be included in a baby's diet. Such nutrients may be far more important than is now realized.

Minimum versus optimum amounts. What shall be our attitude toward the amounts of nutrients to give our babies? Shall we be satisfied with the minimum amount which can give a child the appearance of health, or do we wish to give a more generous amount which may help to build a higher degree of health? For example, most pediatricians believe that 50 milligrams of vitamin C daily is adequate for an infant; yet it is known that under many circumstances the need for this vitamin is tremendously increased (pp. 204, 205, 230). There is much evidence that many nutrients are beneficial when given in what is now considered to be more than adequate amounts. If a generous quantity may help to build a higher degree of health than can a minimum amount, if an excess is not harmful, and if the nutrient can be given without upsetting a baby, it may be wise to err on the side of giving slightly too much rather than too little. Because of this reasoning, I recommend somewhat larger amounts of certain nutrients than do many excellent pediatricians.

The baby's supply of vitamin A. The amount of vitamin A supplied by milk and the cod-liver oil customarily given to infants is considered adequate. Regardless of how perfect the mother's diet may have been during her pregnancy, however, an infant is born poor in the vitamins which dissolve in fat: vitamins A, D, E, and K. Dr. Moore [1] studied the amounts of vitamin A in the bodies of infants who had died from various causes. He found that young infants stored extremely small amounts of this vitamin and that the mucous membranes of their lungs, sinuses and middle ears showed changes typical of vitamin-A deficiency. Such changes are known to predispose an infant to infections. Dr. Wolbach of Harvard University Medical School points out that the inability of the infant to store vitamin A before birth is probably responsible for the fact that babies are particularly susceptible to skin rashes and to such infections as bronchitis, pneumonia, and impetigo. Since an excess of vitamin A can be stored and is not toxic unless millions of units are obtained daily, it seems wiser to give rather generous amounts.

The richest natural source of vitamin A is plain halibut-liver

[1] T. Moore, "The Vitamin A Reserve of the Human Being in Health and Disease," *Biochemical Journal*, 31 (1937), 155.

oil without the addition of viosterol, or vitamin D. This product is available at most drugstores. I have daily given 10 or 20 drops of halibut-liver oil in addition to cod-liver-oil concentrate to our son and have recommended it for years. The halibut-liver oil to which viosterol has been added is designed to be used instead of a cod-liver-oil concentrate and should not be given in addition to it because the combined amounts of vitamin D may be excessive.

Vitamins A and D can be separated from fish-liver oils and put into certain substances which cause them to dissolve readily in water. Preparations of vitamin A alone or both vitamins A and D in aqueous solution are available and appear to have many advantages over the fish-liver oils. These vitamins in water are absorbed more completely into the blood than are those in oil. Animals given these preparations store far larger amounts of the vitamin than when receiving the same number of units dissolved in fat. Drops of the solutions can be added directly to a formula without fear that the vitamins will adhere to the bottles. If the child spits up, only a small amount of the vitamins are lost compared with perhaps the entire quantity when a cod-liver-oil concentrate is given. The danger of the baby's choking is also eliminated. Since these preparations are practically tasteless, they can be mixed with juices, milk, cereals, or any food to be given an older child. The dosage ranges from 3 to 5 drops daily. I changed to these preparations * in feeding our little girl mostly because I found it easier to add them to her formula than to remember to give her drops of fish-liver-oil concentrates after a feeding.

Babies given the B vitamins are easy to care for. With the exception of vitamin B_2 in cows' milk, neither breast milk nor cows' milk is a good source of the B vitamins. The infant's need for the B vitamins has long been recognized, and cereals have been introduced earlier and earlier to supply these vitamins. The facts remain, however, that an infant should receive adequate B

* Aquasol A Drops and Aquasol A and D Drops, U. S. Vitamin Corporation, Casimir Funk Laboratories, New York, N. Y. Similar products put out by other companies are probably equally good.

vitamins daily from birth until solid foods can be given, and that most babies cannot eat enough cereal to meet their needs.

Many pediatricians recommend that a baby be given some preparation supplying five of the B vitamins: vitamin B_1, B_2, and B_6, niacin, and pantothenic acid. Anemias occurring in infants, however, have been successfully treated with the two B vitamins: folic acid and vitamin B_{12}. A certain type of infant eczema has been cleared up by giving another B vitamin, biotin. Deficiencies of the B vitamin, para aminobenzoic acid, have been produced in babies by sulfa drugs and corrected by giving the vitamin. Such findings suggest that an infant benefits by receiving all the B vitamins. Furthermore, much evidence indicates that the giving of any one B vitamin increases the need for other B vitamins. The only way all of these vitamins can be supplied is by natural foods or concentrates of these foods. Powdered or concentrated liver, wheat germ in the form of flour, and rice polishings, all rich sources of these vitamins, have been used in feeding young infants, but for one reason or another they are usually not satisfactory. The best food to supply the B vitamins for an infant is powdered brewers' yeast.

For several years I planned diets for the patients of three obstetricians. These women were sent to me each month during their pregnancy. Many became personal friends, and dozens returned to show me their babies. Most of the babies were under the care of an excellent pediatrician who asked the mothers to add brewers' yeast to each bottle of formula; his babies were outstandingly healthy. At the same time, one of the obstetricians whose patients I saw had a large practice among women of the Christian Science faith; these women preferred to come to me for help in feeding their babies rather than to a pediatrician. I started asking these mothers to add yeast to their infants' formulas or drinking water. Since that time almost all the babies brought to me for nutritional guidance have been given brewers' yeast.

I have never known an infant to be upset by yeast provided it was introduced in small amounts and increased gradually (p. 133). I have never known of any baby receiving yeast daily who suffered from constipation, noninfectious diarrhea, poor appetite, eczema, or colic. The main advantage, however, in giving an infant yeast is the mother's. Yeast-fed babies are happy and contented, sleep soundly, cry little, gain readily, and are so extremely healthy that they are easy to care for. The mother can, therefore, enjoy her motherhood.

Brewers' yeast is sold at drugstores and, less expensively, at health-food stores. It is pasteurized and sterile, need not be refrigerated, and can be obtained so finely ground that it rarely plugs the nipple holes. At least I have had no trouble in using nine different types of nipples without the holes being enlarged. If the drinking water or formula is prepared in advance, the B vitamins soak out of the yeast and can be obtained even though some yeast remains in the bottle.

When yeast is used as the main source of B vitamins, the quantity desirable varies with each baby: 1 or 2 level teaspoons is about as much as can be mixed with the amount of drinking water a breast-fed baby will take; 1 or 2 level tablespoons daily, or 1 teaspoon per bottle, usually appears to be sufficient for an artificially fed infant. If yeast tablets are used, this amount is equivalent to 10 tablets per bottle. When 2 tablespoons or more of yeast are given, a circle of yellow pigment can sometimes be noticed on the diapers; this color is vitamin B_2, or riboflavin, and probably indicates that more yeast is being given than is needed.

Bakers' yeast, or live yeast, which grows in the intestinal tract and prevents B vitamins from being absorbed into the blood, should never be given to an infant or an adult.

Why the baby should have orange juice. One of the greatest advances in infant feeding was made when it became customary to give all babies fresh orange juice, rich in vitamins C and P. If the mother's diet has been good, the amount of vitamin C in the infant's blood at birth is so high that his tissues are saturated with the vitamin, a condition considered ideal. Since vitamin C (and also P) cannot be stored in the body, the amount of this vitamin in the blood falls to an undesirable low level within 3 or 4 days unless the baby is fed breast milk of high quality or vitamin C is immediately added to his formula or orange juice is given him daily from birth.

Vitamin C appears to have a number of functions in the body. It is essential to the formation of the cartilagelike base of the bones and teeth; it helps to protect the body from the harmful effects of bacteria, virus, antigens (which cause allergies), certain drugs (p. 207), and a variety of poisons; it is necessary for the utilization of several essential amino acids; unless adequate vitamin C is supplied daily, these valuable building materials cannot be transformed into body tissue. A sufficient amount of this vitamin, therefore, is needed by the infant every day from birth on and particularly during the early weeks when growth is rapid and there has not yet been time to build up the baby's resistance to infections.

Dr. Jeans,[2] professor of pediatrics at the University of Iowa School of Medicine, stresses that the custom of delaying the giving of vitamin C is altogether too common, and even when the orange juice is given, the amounts are much too small to meet the need. Furthermore, orange juice is usually diluted so much that the infant may not be able to take even the small amount offered. Since the juice is already 90 per cent water, why dilute it? Mothers frequently heat the juice slightly, causing a rapid destruction of vitamin C; a lack of the vitamin can be definitely harmful, whereas a little cool liquid, which will quickly heat to body temperature, cannot be.

"In the private practice of medicine," writes Dr. Jeans, "intolerance of orange juice is encountered frequently, but in hospital practice this condition is found most rarely. From the point of view of digestion, orange juice . . . should not disturb the alimentary tract of the most delicate infant." Such intolerance usually means that the infant has thrown up the juice, probably caused by nipple holes being made too large (p. 126). Because of the frequency of reported intolerance, however, pediatricians often recommend that tablets or a liquid supplying synthetic

---

[2] P. C. Jeans, "Feeding of Healthy Infants and Children," *J. Am. Med. Assn.*, **142** (1950), 806.

vitamin C (ascorbic acid) be added to the formula or drinking water. To use the pure vitamin is easier, and larger amounts can be given than could be obtained from orange juice. The synthetic product, however, lacks vitamin P and the minerals supplied by the juice.

Is vitamin P beneficial to an infant? Almost no consideration has been given vitamin P as a nutrient desirable in feeding babies. In correcting vitamin-C deficiencies in infants, however, consistently better results have been obtained by giving orange juice than the synthetic vitamin (ref. 3, p. 85), presumably because of the vitamin P supplied. Vitamin C is better utilized and smaller amounts are needed when vitamin P is given with it. When vitamin P is undersupplied, the walls of the blood vessels become so porous that red corpuscles pass into the tissues, causing the flesh to have a speckled, turkey-egg appearance. These spots, like miniature bruises, are most often seen on the legs.

A few years ago I saw a 4-month-old, bottle-fed infant whose legs were covered with tiny red spots. He had never been given orange juice but only the pure vitamin C. I referred the case to a physician who had done years of research on vitamin P. He told me that the condition was caused by a deficiency of this nutrient and that he frequently saw such infants. When the baby was given vitamin P in the form of sweetened lemon juice and an extract made of the white part of lemon rind (p. 238), the condition cleared up and did not recur. Since that time I have seen three other bottle-fed babies with vitamin-P deficiencies; none of them had been given orange juice.

Cows' milk lacks vitamin P. The amount in breast milk apparently varies with the diet of the mother. The richest sources of vitamin P are the white part of lemon rind and juices of oranges, lemons, and black currants.[3] Grapefruit, prune, and grape juices are fair sources. Although many books on baby feeding recommend that either orange or tomato juice be given an

[3] A. L. Bacharach and M. E. Coates, "The Vitamin P Activity of Fruits and Vegetables," *Journal of the Society of the Chemical Industry,* **62** (1943), 85.

infant, tomato juice contains little vitamin P and is un
as a source of vitamin C; if it is given, it should be in
citrus juice. Since vitamin P is little harmed by cannin,
ing, canned or frozen citrus juices may be used as a source of this
nutrient. These juices vary in their content of vitamin C, but some
are so carefully prepared that they contain as much of the vitamin
as does freshly squeezed juice, which averages 15 milligrams of
vitamin C per ounce.

In order that an infant obtain both vitamins C and P, it is
probably wise to give him 1 ounce of undiluted orange juice daily
as soon as he is home from the hospital; this amount should be
doubled when the juice is seen to be well tolerated. By the time
the baby is 1 month old, the juice could be further increased to
3 ounces daily and to 4 and 5 ounces when he is 3 and 4 months
old, respectively. A bottle-fed baby, however, would still not
obtain enough vitamin C to promote ideal health; a tablet or
liquid supplying at least 50 milligrams of the pure vitamin should
be added to his formula.

The importance of vitamin D cannot be overemphasized.
Vitamin D is so important that Chapter 19 is devoted largely to
the subject (p. 210). Neither breast milk nor cows' milk supplies
enough of this nutrient to promote health. Although the vitamin
D added to evaporated milk is valuable, it is insufficient to meet
the needs in an infant who eats little or grows rapidly. The cod-
liver oil, cod-liver-oil concentrate, vitamin D in aqueous solution,
or a similar preparation recommended by your pediatrician will
probably be the only dependable source of this vitamin your baby
will obtain.

Studies have shown that babies given adequate vitamin D will
store 60 to 80 per cent of the calcium obtained, whereas if no
vitamin D is given, 90 to 100 per cent of the calcium ingested is
lost in the feces. Similarly four or five times more phosphorus is
usually retained when vitamin D is adequate than when it is not
supplied. Bones cannot develop normally unless these valuable
minerals are held in the body.

Since it is difficult to give 1 teaspoon or more of cod-liver oil to a young infant without causing him to choke, most pediatricians recommend that 5 or 10 drops of a cod-liver-oil concentrate or some similar preparation be given. Whenever an oil is used, the drops should be put directly on the infant's tongue, *never into a bottle*. Preparations of vitamins A and D in aqueous solution (p. 94), however, mix readily with milk and can be added to the formula or drinking water.

Should your baby be given vitamin E and unsaturated fatty acids? At the present time, neither vitamin E nor unsaturated fatty acids are considered essential nutrients in the feeding of infants. Average breast milk, however, contains ten times more vitamin E than does cows' milk and is a far richer source of these essential acids. Although no one knows why breast milk should be so rich in these nutrients, nature may have put them there for a designed purpose.

Experiments have shown that less vitamin A is destroyed in the body and smaller amounts are needed when vitamin E is generously supplied. If the young of almost any animal is deficient in vitamin E, its muscles fail to develop normally; similar failure in muscular development (muscular dystrophy) in children has sometimes been treated successfully with vitamin E. Babies with poorly developed muscles are all too common, and it is possible, though unproved, that a lack of vitamin E is responsible.

Until vitamin E is proved to be unnecessary to the health of babies, it seems wise to give this vitamin to the bottle-fed infant. The richest natural source of vitamin E is wheat-germ oil, sold inexpensively at drugstores and health-food stores. For years I have recommended that mothers of bottle-fed babies give them daily 10 drops or more of wheat-germ oil. Like other vitamins in oil, it should be put directly on the tongue, not into the formula. Since the B vitamins do not dissolve in fat, wheat-germ oil must never be considered a source of B vitamins even though wheat germ itself contains them.

Butter fat and cod-liver oil appear to be almost completely

lacking in the essential unsaturated fatty acids found principally in vegetable oils. Since these acids are destroyed in making margarine, the bottle-fed baby usually receives little or none of them until he is old enough to eat salads. When infants, suffering from a certain type of eczema, are given unsaturated fatty acids, the eczema disappears.[4] These nutrients, therefore, appear to be beneficial. Since wheat-germ oil is about 50 per cent essential unsaturated fatty acids, if it is given as a source of vitamin E, these acids are supplied in an amount comparable to that obtained by the breast-fed baby. Since oils can be absorbed through the skin, rubbing a baby with corn or soybean oil rather than the questionable mineral oil (p. 160) may be another means of supplying these acids.

Give vitamins in oil after a feeding. When vitamins A, D, and E are given in oil, they are carried through the intestinal wall into the blood only after they have combined with bile salts. Since little bile flows into the intestine except after a meal, it is extremely important that these vitamins be given·an infant only after a feeding. The oils supplying these vitamins may be given immediately after the baby has been thoroughly burped or within ½ hour after he has been fed.

The best time to give these vitamins is after the first feeding in the morning. The infant is less likely to go to sleep after this feeding than after later meals. Furthermore, in case the mother forgets to give the oils, she may remember them after a later feeding; if she waits until the evening feeding and then forgets them, the infant misses his quota of these vitamins for the day.

When cod-liver-oil concentrate, wheat-germ oil, and plain halibut-liver oil are used, all three oils may be given after the same feeding. In fact, equal amounts of the three oils can be combined, and 30 drops of the mixture given rather than 10 drops of each. When the infant is only a few days old, however, it is advisable

[4] A. E. Hansen, "Serum Lipid Changes and Therapeutic Effects of Various Oils in Infantile Eczema," *Proceedings of the Society of Experimental Biology and Medicine,* 31 (1933), 160; "Serum Lipids in Eczema," *Am. J. Dis. Child.,* 53 (1937), 933.

to give him no more than 5 drops of oil at a time and allow him to swallow before more is offered him.

Should vitamin K ever be given as a supplement? Vitamin K is necessary before a substance, prothrombin, can be formed; prothrombin, in turn, is essential to the clotting of blood. Apparently all newborn infants suffer from a deficiency of this vitamin, causing them to hemorrhage so readily that most obstetricians now give injections of vitamin K to the baby soon after birth. Since some obstetricians, however, do not give this vitamin, a lack of it may prove tragic.

Studies have shown that the greatest number of hemorrhages occur on the sixth day after birth but that the clotting time may remain dangerously slow for the first 2 weeks; that the ability of the blood to clot increases gradually but does not become normal until a baby is about 10 months old (ref. 2, p. 39). Although the hemorrhages occurring in the brain and spinal cord have the most serious consequences for the babies who survive them, bleeding throughout the body is common; it may occur from the navel, mouth, nose, ears, pelvis or vagina, or the intestinal tract, as is shown by black, tarry stools.

Cows' milk contains almost no vitamin K in comparison with breast milk, which is often a rich source. Thus the breast-fed baby usually gets this vitamin at each feeding, whereas the artificially fed baby is lucky to get one injection of it at birth. The bottle-fed baby might well benefit by having 1 milligram of this vitamin added to his daily formula, at least during the first 3 weeks. The cost would be about 10 cents and might prevent the expenditure of thousands of dollars.

Before leaving the hospital, find out whether your obstetrician gave your baby vitamin K. If any evidence of bleeding should occur, call your pediatrician immediately. In case your tiny son is to be circumcised when he is only a few days old, or if any other surgery is undertaken, make sure that he receives some form of vitamin K first.

Your baby's need for iron, copper, and iodine. Although average breast milk contains twice as much iron and a third more copper than does cows' milk, neither type of milk is a good source of these minerals. If the mother's prenatal diet was adequate, enough iron and copper are stored by a full-term infant to prevent anemia for a few months. It is generally believed, however, that foods rich in iron should be supplied an infant as soon as possible.

If vegetables, lightly salted with iodized salt, are cooked in a small amount of water and that water is given to a baby to drink or is added to his formula, significant quantities of iron, copper, and iodine are supplied. An excellent source of iron and copper for infants is blackstrap molasses; 1 teaspoon of this molasses furnishes more than 3 milligrams of iron, or twice the amount supplied by an egg yolk. This molasses is so laxative that no more than ⅓ teaspoon should be added to the formula or drinking water until it is seen to be well tolerated.

If you live in the Middle West or the Pacific Northwest, where the soil and water are known to be deficient in iodine, it is undoubtedly wise to purchase a thin solution of iodine, such as Lugol's solution, and add 3 or 4 drops daily to your baby's formula or drinking water. The mother of a breast-fed infant would do well to take Lugol's solution herself and thus assure that her milk would supply her infant's needs.

Supplements are particularly important for the premature infant. Compared with babies born at term, premature infants are nutritionally handicapped. These babies store almost no vitamin A. Since vitamin C is necessary for the utilization of several essential amino acids, tiny infants require this vitamin in greater quantities than do larger babies, and the need exists almost immediately after birth. It has long been known that premature infants are particularly susceptible to rickets. Their lack of vitamin K is so marked that their blood often contains only 3 per cent of the normal amount of prothrombin; hemorrhages are frequent and cause many such infants to die during or soon after birth. So little iron, calcium, and phosphorus are stored in their bodies before birth that anemia and faulty bone structure are the rule rather than the exception.

Premature infants, whose requirements are thus unusually high, are able to drink less milk than can larger babies. Their mothers are more often unable to nurse them; hence they cannot obtain the nutrients supplied more generously in breast milk than in cows' milk. It becomes particularly important, therefore, that adequate amounts of nutritional supplements be given the premature infant and that they be started 3 or 4 days after birth.

The belief is widely held that babies born prematurely need larger amounts of vitamin D than do infants born at term. Recent studies [5] have shown, however, that the bones of premature infants fail to develop normally because such infants have stored so little minerals before birth and because they can drink such small quantities of milk that they obtain too little calcium and phosphorus to build normal bones. The time may soon come when pediatricians, instead of advising larger amounts of vitamin D, will ask the mother to add perhaps ⅛ teaspoon of some calcium salt, such as calcium gluconate, to each bottle of formula for the premature baby.

The amount of each supplement recommended for full-term babies is probably adequate for premature infants provided the supplements are started during the first few days of life and given daily thereafter.

Too little, too late. Mothers, particularly young mothers with their first babies, are often afraid that a baby will be upset by being given a few drops of fish-liver-oil concentrate or a little yeast or molasses. They are frequently hesitant to start orange juice for fear the baby will develop an allergy to it. Usually the smaller the baby, the greater the fear. It is extremely important for the mother to realize that her baby may need the supplement far more during the second or third week of life than during the second or third month.

There is one rule which should always be followed in feeding a baby: introduce any food or supplement in only a small amount

[5] K. Glaser, A. H. Parmelee, and W. S. Hoffman, "Comparative Efficacy of Vitamin D Preparations in Prophylactic Treatment of Premature Infants," *Am. J. Dis. Child.*, **77** (1949), 1.

at first. A small quantity cannot upset an infant, whereas a larger one might. The amount of fat in 5 or 10 drops of cod-liver-oil concentrate, halibut-liver oil, and wheat-germ oil, or protein in a little yeast, or of sugar in ¼ teaspoon of molasses is small indeed in comparison with the quantity of fat, protein, and sugar a newborn baby obtains from milk. It is unlikely any of these foods could upset the most delicate stomach. Strained orange juice is little more than sugar (glucose) and water, extremely similar to the glucose and water given to most babies before the mother's milk comes in.

My attitude, therefore, is exactly opposite to that of many mothers: instead of being afraid to give supplements, I would be ten times more afraid not to give them; the smaller the baby, the more afraid I would be to delay the supplements. Giving supplements rarely causes harm; delaying them often causes serious and irreparable damage.

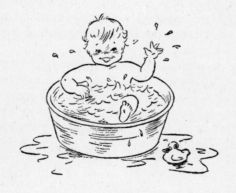

CHAPTER 10

FORMULAS FOR MOTHERS
OF BOTTLE-FED BABIES

IF A mother secretes enough milk to nurse her baby, she must stay on a fairly adequate diet; otherwise the milk will dry up. The mother who gives her baby a formula can and usually does commit dietary crimes against herself for which she is quickly and severely punished. The punishment takes the form of torturing fatigue, jumpy nerves, irritability, a haggard appearance, excessive worrying, mental depression, and, not infrequently, uncontrollable sobbing.

The fact that a mother cannot produce sufficient milk usually indicates that her diet during pregnancy has been faulty. Without realizing it, she may already be suffering from multiple deficiencies. Perhaps her delivery has been difficult, and she still feels ill. Perhaps she has to get up twice or three times each night to care for her baby. Perhaps the older children are suddenly acting like little fiends, soiling their panties, demanding bottles, and claiming their mother's time and attention in every possible way. The books on psychology have forewarned her, but an exhausted mother is rarely an expert in applied psychology. As the yelling of the older children grates on her shattered nerves, more than one well-bred mother has found herself returning yell for yell. She may have little or no time to prepare or eat breakfast or lunch; she gulps cups of coffee (oh, for a whole night of uninterrupted sleep!) and grabs perhaps cookies or doughnuts; by dinnertime she is too tired to care. A vicious circle is formed.

A pediatrician will work out a formula for the baby, but no one guides the mother's health. Usually she needs help far more than does the baby. The trouble is that the more her diet needs improving, the harder it is for her to improve it because of fatigue and mental confusion.

The B vitamins are a "must." Let us, then, start with mere essentials, the "musts." Whenever you miss sleep and/or increase the amount of work you do, your need for those hard-to-get B vitamins increases. The lack of B vitamins causes immediate fatigue. Time and again scientists have kept volunteers on a diet adequate in all respects except one of the B vitamins. In such experiments, whether the missing nutrient is vitamin B_1 or B_6, niacin or biotin, the resulting symptoms are the same: not only fatigue and decreased endurance, but also the blue-Monday blues, irritability, tendency to worry, slowed and confused thinking, an I-can't-take-it-another-minute feeling, and often an uncontrollable desire to cry without knowing why. The symptoms are the same as those experienced time and again by mothers of new babies. The reason they are the same is that the causes are the same.

If you are to feel well, you must get as many foods rich in all the B vitamins as you can. The only really good sources are liver, brewers' yeast, and wheat germ. Since the amount of vitamins in 1 heaping tablespoon of yeast roughly equals the quantity in a serving of liver (¼ pound) or ½ cup of wheat germ, yeast is the most convenient even though you may dislike it at first. If you can take 1 heaping tablespoon daily, chances are you will experience a noticeable lift. By the time you have increased the amount to 2 heaping tablespoons daily, you will probably feel on top of the world. When you begin taking 3 tablespoons daily, you may find yourself working twice as hard without tiring.

Add wheat germ to your breakfast cereal or use it as a cold cereal or have wheat germ and middlings as a cooked cereal. If you feel life is hardly worth living, try to eat liver daily for a while; at least have liverwurst for lunch. Use yogurt and black-strap molasses as additional sources of B vitamins as often as you can. Sprinkle the yogurt well with cinnamon and sweeten it with blackstrap; or stir the molasses into milk or take it directly from a spoon. Every time you find your usual self-confidence being crowded out by worry that your baby may die with each squirm, wiggle, or sneeze, increase your intake of B vitamins still more. Further information concerning foods rich in these vitamins is found on pages 29 and 262.

A good breakfast is essential to well-being. The second "must" is a good breakfast. Regardless of how much you may skimp on your other meals, do not miss breakfast if you want to feel well during the day. A dozen or more studies have been made at various universities showing that your efficiency and feeling of well-being depend more on a good breakfast than on any other meal. At the University of Iowa,[1] for example, young women were found to be less nervous, to think more quickly, and to work harder without fatigue when they ate a breakfast of fruit or juice, cereal, buttered toast, and milk than when they went without breakfasts or drank unsweetened black coffee. Although they ate breakfasts of 300, 600, and 1,000 calories over different periods, none of the girls gained weight even on the largest breakfast. Apparently they felt so much better after eating the large breakfast that they unconsciously used the extra calories in greater energy output. In still another study [2] persons were found to be more energetic throughout the day and to experience the greatest sense of well-being when their breakfasts were high in protein (20 grams or more [p. 24]); also the amount of sugar in their blood remained high for the longest period.

Watch that coffee-pot. If you are particularly tired and sleepy, you may be relying on frequent cups of coffee for a pickup. Try to cut down your amount of coffee drinking as quickly as you feel good enough to do so. The Iowa study showed that the girls could do less work and suffered greater nervousness

[1] K. Daum, W. W. Tuttle, C. Martin, and L. Myers, "Effect of Various Breakfasts on Physiologic Response," *Am. J. Diet. Assn.*, 26 (1950), 503.

[2] E. Orent-Keiles and L. F. Hallman, "The Breakfast Meal in Relation to Blood Sugar Values," *U. S. Department of Agriculture,* Circular No. 827 (1949).

when their breakfast consisted only of coffee than when they went without breakfast; that they improved when breakfast was eaten with coffee, but were more efficient when the only beverage was milk. Experiments conducted at the University of Wisconsin showed that well-fed animals, given coffee, developed symptoms of multiple B-vitamin deficiencies, including rapid aging and the graying of hair; injections of caffeine alone had no effect. It is possible that coffee may cause a similar loss or destruction of B vitamins in the human body.

Keep your other meals simple. If you can manage to take 2 or 3 tablespoons of yeast daily and to eat a hearty breakfast, you will probably find yourself feeling so well that it is no longer a chore to prepare and eat the other meals. Regardless of how busy you are, try to get adequate protein. Make your daily goal 1 quart of whole or skim milk or buttermilk; an egg; a serving each of cheese and meat. Do not feel that you must take time to cook. When you are too busy to prepare lunch, grab a piece of cheese or some cold meats or hot dogs, 1 or 2 glasses of milk and some fruit; place the food within reach and eat it as you feed the baby, propping the bottle neatly between the buttons of a blouse which opens down the front. Plan dinners of easy-to-cook foods: chops or ground-meat patties, a thawed vegetable, a raw vegetable or salad, milk, and fruit for dessert. Dinners should be filling but light so that the entire family will be hungry for a large breakfast.

Since your diet must supply all known nutrients if health is to be maintained, depend on vitamin capsules or tablets to furnish the nutrients you are too busy to get in your foods. If you have no time to prepare or eat colored fruits and vegetables, take a capsule containing 10,000 units or more of vitamin A and some vitamin D. If you have no time to squeeze fresh orange juice, drink canned or frozen juice; if you fail in that, take a vitamin-C tablet daily. Eat enough wheat germ to supply some vitamin E. Ample calcium will be furnished by the milk; iron, phosphorus, and other minerals, by the proteins and foods rich in B vitamins.

Such a diet would be far from perfect, but it will keep you from feeling you have reached the end of your rope.

Drying up milk. Physicians must sometimes recommend that women should not nurse their babies. To dry up their milk as quickly as possible, these women often eat little protein and keep their liquid intake to a minimum. In many cases, their diets are already deficient in protein, the B vitamins, and many other nutrients. Their health may have been severely taxed by their pregnancies. Many of them, particularly the mothers with several young children, must work harder and for longer hours on less sleep than ever before. Under such circumstances fatigue, irritability, crying spells, and excessive worrying are inevitable.

When breasts are bound and not completely emptied, milk quickly dries up. Whenever necessary, express enough milk to relieve discomfort. Stay on the best diet possible so that you can cope with the increased amount of work and lack of sleep without undue fatigue. To eat an inadequate diet purposely at a time when your nutritional needs have skyrocketed, however, is a matter to consider seriously. Realize that it cannot be done without severe penalty.

If you put yourself on a good "formula" first, your baby's formula will probably cause you few worries.

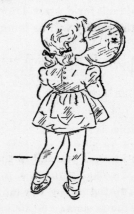

CHAPTER 11

THE REQUIREMENTS
OF A GOOD FORMULA

NURSING a baby appears to be best for his psychological development. Since the quality of breast milk, however, depends on the diet of the mother, it is possible to construct formulas superior to certain breast milks. If you hold your baby while you feed him, his psychological needs can also be met. Let us now see if a standard formula can meet his physiological needs.

How standard formulas are constructed. Since breast milk differs considerably from cows' milk, in making a formula cows' milk is usually altered so that it is as nearly like breast milk as possible. The approximate composition in per cent of the two types of milk is as follows:

Type of Milk	Fat	Sugar	Protein	Total Minerals
Human	3.5	7.5	1.25	0.20
Cows'	3.5	4.7	3.4	0.75

When cows' milk is diluted with water, its protein and mineral content is decreased; then if a certain amount of sugar is added, the resulting formula is similar in composition to breast milk. Although this procedure has been accepted for years, it is now argued that such formulas can be improved upon.

A baby needs protein for growth. All growth depends upon an adequate supply of protein; an infant grows more rapidly than at any other time during life; hence his need for protein is greater than it will ever be again. Dr. Jeans (ref. 2, p. 97) points out that artificially fed babies receiving protein equivalent to that of breast milk have poorer tissue turgor and motor development than do babies given more protein or less diluted cows' milk. Many studies have been made in which already digested proteins, or protein hydrolysates, have been added to infants' formulas, thus making the food far richer in protein than is breast milk. These studies have consistently shown that infants given more protein thrive better than do babies fed the usual formulas.

Another way to construct a formula higher than usual in protein is to make it of undiluted fresh cows' milk or of evaporated milk diluted with an equal amount of water. This procedure was followed in a study made by Dr. Gordon and Dr. Levine.[1] Since premature infants are more difficult to feed than are full-term babies, these doctors selected premature infants for their study. They divided the babies into three groups and gave all of them food containing the same number of calories. Protein supplied 7 per cent of the calories for one group given breast milk or formulas of diluted milk. Another group, fed evaporated milk diluted with an equal amount of water, received 16 per cent of their calories in the form of protein. A third group, given undiluted cows' milk with half of the cream poured off, received 20 per cent of their calories as protein; thus they obtained almost three times as much protein as did the babies receiving breast milk.

The infants given the largest amount of protein thrived far better than did the others. The babies weighing the least at birth made the most spectacular gains and were able to leave the hospital sooner than did larger babies receiving less protein. All the infants in the two high-protein groups tolerated the formulas better than did infants fed smaller amounts of protein. Such a study indicates that it may be desirable to give bottle-fed babies more protein than they would receive in formulas simulating breast milk.

Although such formulas may seem concentrated, it is well to

[1] H. H. Gordon and S. Z. Levine, "Feeding of Premature Infants, a Comparison of Human Milk and Cows' Milk," *Am. J. Dis. Child.*, 73 (1947), 442.

remember that colostrum, or a mother's first milk, often contains almost twice as much protein as does undiluted cows' milk.

Too much sugar may be detrimental. Another argument against standard formulas is that the amount of sugar equivalent to that in breast milk is more than is needed. Sugar is used principally to produce energy; if not required for energy, it is converted into fat. A healthy, well-fed baby is not especially energetic; he sleeps most of the time. Although a certain amount of stored fat is desirable, it is far more important that a gain in weight represent increased body structures such as new muscle tissue, normal bone development, and greater blood volume instead of an increase of stored fat. Sugar cannot aid growth in any way; it cannot build blood, muscles, teeth, bones, hormones, antibodies, or any tissues vital to health.

Another reason why it seems unwise to add much sugar to a formula is that certain B vitamins are necessary before sugar can be converted into energy or stored as fat. The higher the sugar content of the formula, the greater the need for adequate amounts of these vitamins, which are only meagerly supplied by either breast or cows' milk. The addition of sugar beyond that actually needed can cause symptoms of B-vitamin deficiencies to appear. Although not all pediatricians would agree, colic appears to be nothing more than gas pains caused by the fermentation of sugar in the intestines, resulting from a multiple B-vitamin deficiency which has allowed digestion and absorption to become faulty.

Another argument against adding much sugar to a formula is that artificially fed babies are inclined to get too fat, whereas breast-fed infants rarely do although they receive more fat and the same amount of sugar. Excessive fat can be prevented if less sugar is added to the formula. Dr. Holt,[2] professor of pediatrics at New York University Medical School, points out that fat babies are much more subject to chafing, eczema, allergies, and infections of the skin than are babies who are less fat.

The type of sugar used in formulas has also been criticized.

[2] L. E. Holt, Jr., "Dietary Requirements During the First Two Years of Life," *Clinical Proceedings of Children's Hospital,* **2** (1946), 251.

The only sugar found in any kind of milk is milk sugar, or lactose. This sugar is not particularly sweet. Instead of using milk sugar entirely for formulas, however, table sugar, corn syrup, or a mixture of two sugars, dextrose (grape sugar) and maltose (malt sugar), are more often used. Since these sugars are much sweeter, it is argued that babies are trained from birth to enjoy excessively sweet foods, making them crave sweets later and causing them to eat far too many candies, cookies, and desserts. Oversweet formulas may thus be partly responsible for the rampant tooth decay and other manifestations of inferior health all too common today.

Another argument for using milk sugar in an infant's formula is that it supports the growth of millions of desirable bacteria in the intestine, whereas other sugars do not (ref. 2, p. 113). These bacteria, for example, produce vitamin K; the bottle-fed infant may not obtain this life-saving nutrient from another source for many weeks; when sugars which cannot support bacterial growth are used, the baby may not even obtain vitamin K from bacterial synthesis. Intestinal bacteria also synthesize certain of the B vitamins and perhaps all of them. Breast milk is low in these vitamins probably because nature intended the intestinal bacteria supported by milk sugar to supply them.

A third argument for using milk sugar in a formula is that part of this sugar is changed by intestinal bacteria into lactic acid. Vitamin C and several of the B vitamins are readily destroyed in the body unless they are held in acid until they reach the blood. Furthermore, calcium, phosphorus, iron, and many essential minerals can dissolve only in acid; unless dissolved, they cannot be absorbed. Because of the greater amount of lactic acid produced by bacteria in the intestines of the baby who is nursed, the infant absorbs far more calcium and iron from breast milk than from a standard formula supplying the same amounts of these minerals.

Breast milk probably contains so much sugar for three reasons: first, to support the growth of valuable bacteria; second, to permit conversion of much of the milk sugar by bacteria into lactic acid, thus protecting many of the vitamins and facilitating the efficient absorption of minerals; and third, to assure the production of vitamin K and the B vitamins by the bacteria living on the sugar. Only a small proportion of the sugar in breast milk may be left for the baby to use for energy or store as fat; thus the breast-fed baby does not become sloppy fat as do thousands of infants given standard formulas containing the same amount of sugar but of a different kind.

The sweeter sugars used in infants' formulas cannot be converted into lactic acid. On the contrary, they stimulate the flow of alkaline digestive juices in the intestine. Thus they probably allow the destruction of certain vitamins and interfere with the absorption of iron, calcium, and phosphorus to such an extent that they can be detrimental to the development of the blood, bones, and teeth. Since these sugars are little needed to produce energy, they are converted into useless and unsightly fat.

Two conclusions, therefore, appear to be justified: that a formula need not contain as much sugar as does breast milk; and that milk sugar is preferable to other sugars for a baby.

Do standard formulas supply an ideal amount of fat? Breast milk and undiluted cows' milk contain the same amount of fat, whereas the usual formula contains only about half as much. Dr. Holt (ref. 2, p. 113) points out that babies who receive diets low in fat are particularly susceptible to skin infections and eczema even though all known vitamins are generously supplied. He cites a case of a baby who developed eczema and asthma every time fat was withdrawn from the diet; yet both abnormalities disappeared as soon as fat was again given. It is possible that the small amount of fat in the standard formula may be partly responsible for the fact that the bottle-fed baby is more susceptible to allergies than is the breast-fed infant.

In discussing overweight babies, Dr. Holt states as his belief that the usual procedure of removing the fat from the formula to decrease calories while continuing to add sugar is absolutely wrong. Fat stays in the stomach longer than does protein or sugar and thus prevents hunger pains. Persons "reducing" on fat-free diets usually become so starved that they overeat and gain more than if they had eaten some fat. One reason why breast-fed infants do not become disgustingly fat is probably that the fat they obtain sticks to their ribs, satisfies their hunger, and causes them to consume fewer calories. Contradictory though it may seem, the best way to prevent an infant from becoming over-weight may be to allow him more appetite-satisfying fat than a standard formula supplies.

From a mother's point of view, a baby is much easier to care for when given a formula containing the same amount of fat as that found in breast milk. Such a baby gets hungry less fre-quently and, since his appetite is satisfied, sleeps soundly for long periods; thus the mother has more time for herself.

Pediatricians often hesitate to recommend a formula containing much fat because undigested fat can usually be found in an infant's stools. Recent studies have shown, however, that when the fat content of a formula is doubled or tripled, the propor-tion of fat digested stays approximately the same; thus the infant can absorb two or three times more fat than he could if given a low-fat formula. Furthermore, no harm is done by the fat left undigested.

The ideal formula. When we consider all the objections to the standard formula, we find that an ideal formula should be higher in protein and slightly lower in sugar than is breast milk and the same in fat. If fresh cows' milk is used undiluted or is diluted with only a little water, and if no sugar is added, these standards are met. A formula fulfilling these requirements could also be made of evaporated milk diluted with an equal amount of water or only slightly more water than milk. Such a formula is infinitely easier for a mother to prepare than is a standard formula. Let us now see what results have been obtained when babies have been fed such formulas.

Dr. McCulloch,[3] professor of clinical pediatrics at the Wash-ington University Medical School, has reported the progress of

[3] H. McCulloch, "Use of Evaporated Milk Without Added Sugar for the Feeding of Infants," *Am. J. Dis. Child.*, **67** (1944), 52.

a large number of infants, both premature and full-term, who have been kept on formulas of evaporated milk and water without any added sugar. Whenever the infants were hungry, they were fed; they were allowed to take any amount of formula they desired. These babies stayed in excellent general health. They suffered neither from diarrhea nor constipation but averaged two to four bowel movements daily. They did little spitting up and almost no vomiting. No infant had intestinal gas or gas distension; all were free from colic. They had excellent appetites, developed unusually firm muscle tone, and slept better and for longer periods than do infants given standard formulas.

It is not surprising that Dr. McCulloch recommends formulas without added sugar for all babies, particularly infants suffering from colic or other gastrointestinal disturbances. He points out that added sugar is detrimental to general health; that it produces flabby, overweight babies who are pale and irritable; and that it retards the development of teeth and bones and produces poor muscle tone and low resistance to infections.

Dr. Adams,[4] who had charge of the Pediatrics Department of the Navy Hospital in San Diego during the second world war, is equally enthusiastic about this type of formula. In his study, 56 premature infants and 700 full-term babies were given equal amounts of evaporated milk and water without added sugar. Such formulas, started when the infants were 2 days old, were continued until they were 5 months old, at which time they were put on pasteurized milk.

This doctor states that the formula was used with surprising success. Not one infant of the entire 756 showed any intolerance to the formula. None had colic, diarrhea, or constipation. Bowel movements ranged from one to eight daily, with an average of five. Many babies showed no loss of weight after birth, and most of the others lost less than was expected. The premature infants regained their birth weight earlier and were discharged from the hospital 2 or 3 days sooner than were premature babies who

4 F. H. Adams, "A Simple Formula for Premature and Full Term Infants," *J. Pediat.*, **33** (1948), 23.

were breast fed. Dr. Adams states that they developed better bone structure and firmer muscle tone than babies do when given standard formulas.

A study of 2,004 infants given similar formulas without added sugar is reported by Dr. McMahon,[5] a pediatrician practicing in Milwaukee, Wisconsin. He also found that formulas made of equal parts of evaporated milk and water were far superior to standard formulas; that the infants were freer from vomiting, diarrhea, constipation, colic, and similar disturbances; that their muscle tone and resistance to disease was higher; and that such a formula is so well tolerated that the infants were easy to care for.

Dr. Gerstley[6] and coworkers at the Michael Reese Hospital in Chicago also recommend high-protein formulas with no sugar added, but their reasons are different. They studied the absorption of calcium and phosphorus in infants 3 weeks to 6 months old when given four different formulas. The study showed that the largest amount of these minerals was absorbed and the best bone development resulted when the babies were breast fed or given undiluted cows' milk without added sugar. When fresh milk was diluted and milk sugar added, a smaller quantity of these minerals reached the blood. A formula of diluted cows' milk and dextromaltose caused a marked decrease in the absorption of calcium and phosphorus. When dextromaltose was added to whole milk, so little calcium and phosphorus were absorbed that rickets developed rapidly. The formula was considered so dangerous that this phase of their study was terminated immediately.

These physicians recommend that no sugar be added to a baby's formula; they are convinced that sugar interferes so seriously with the absorption of calcium and phosphorus and is so detrimental to the teeth and bones that they even question the

---

[5] H. O. McMahon, "Report of Use of Evaporated Milk and Water in 2,004 Cases," *Wisconsin Medical Journal*, 38 (1939), 874.

[6] J. R. Gerstley, D. J. Cohn, and G. Lawrence, "A Study of Calcium and Phosphorus Metabolism and of Clinical Findings as Influenced by Certain Feedings," *J. Pediat.*, 27 (1945), 521.

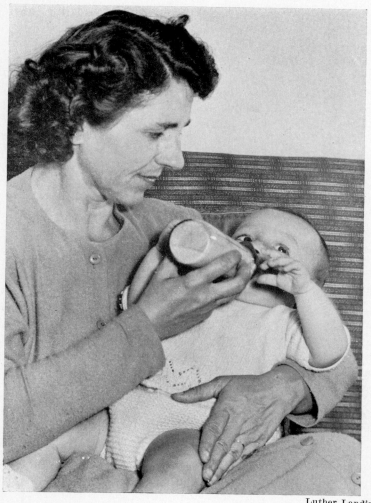

Enjoy holding your baby while you can. Each period of growth is fascinating, but the intimacy and warmth between yourself and your child and the many joys of babyhood can never be recaptured.

wisdom of feeding cereals early. All cereals contain much starch which is changed into sugar during digestion. Actually the formula these doctors considered dangerous is frequently given to babies 4 to 6 months old; it is highly recommended in several recent books on infant feeding.

Such studies indicate that criticism of the standard low-protein, low-fat, high-sugar formulas is justified. Furthermore, these studies show that formulas high in protein and fat but without added sugar offer advantages every mother desires: babies free from colic, healthy, and easy to care for.

Let us now see what kind of milk may be most desirable in making a formula.

Using pasteurized milk for an infant. Pasteurized milk to be given to a young baby must first be boiled. As every housewife knows, milk boils over so quickly that when a formula is made of it, much time must be spent scrubbing the range. My feeling is that the physician who recommends a pasteurized-milk formula has had too few children or has not prepared formulas frequently enough himself.

The scum which forms over boiled milk contains a valuable protein, lactalbumin; when it is removed, much nutritive value is lost. Another disadvantage of using pasteurized milk, collected from many small producers, is that you know nothing of the amount of poison sprays used in the barns or on the food which the cows have eaten. When such poisons are used, a certain amount of them is found in the milk; they may cause your baby to have digestive upsets. The animals' food is often produced on inferior soils under poor agricultural treatment, and the resulting milk is low in nutritive value. Although most states prohibit the sale of milk from diseased cows, the fact remains that such milk is sold. When the cows are examined annually, thousands of diseased animals are weeded out; the milk produced previous to the discovery of the disease is sold. It may be given to your baby.

Most pediatricians consider that by the time a baby is 6 months old, pasteurized milk can safely be given without first being boiled. My advice would be to use some other form of milk for a younger infant.

The advantages of using raw certified milk. From the standpoint of nutrition, raw certified milk appears to be superior to pasteurized or evaporated milk for feeding infants. This milk is produced by bovine aristocracy. Since a certified herd is given the best food available, again and again such milk has been found to have a higher vitamin and mineral content than do other types of milk.

Dr. Francis M. Pottenger [7] has shown that far superior health can be produced in babies given certified raw milk instead of pasteurized or evaporated-milk formulas. Dr. Pottenger's x-rays of the bones of infants fed certified milk are so spectacular compared with those of infants given standard formulas that anyone seeing them would probably never forget them. Excellent skeletal structure is shown not only by the strong white shadows indicating densely mineralized bones but also by the width of the chest, the breadth of the dental arch, and even the thickness of the bones themselves. The bones of the infants given pasteurized or evaporated milk show slight mineral deposits; the chests are narrow, the dental arches underdeveloped, and the bones themselves thin and fragile. It may be well to remember that the fortunate breast-fed infant whose mother consumes an adequate diet receives only "raw certified milk."

We do not know exactly which health-improving nutrients are destroyed by heat during pasteurization or canning. It is known, however, that some of the amino acids from proteins are harmed, particularly by the high heat used when milk is canned; that certain hormones, vitamin B_{12} and the enzyme, phosphatase (which aids in the absorption of phosphorus), are destroyed even by the mild heat used in pasteurizing. It has recently been found that raw milk contains a valuable steroid similar to ACTH. In all probability unknown heat-labile factors

[7] F. M. Pottenger, "Clinical and Experimental Evidence of Growth Factors in Raw Milk," Certified Milk, American Association of Medical Milk Commissions, 1 (1937), 1.

such as antibiotics occur in raw milk, which may aid directly or indirectly in producing health.

Although I knew of the proved superiority of unboiled certified raw milk, I was formerly afraid to use it for feeding infants. When several physicians urged me to give our baby girl certified milk, I discussed the matter with the officials in charge of the production of this milk at our local dairy. They told me that no DDT or other poison sprays were used in the barns where the certified herds were kept; that no poison sprays were allowed to be used on the feed given these animals; that bovine tuberculosis or Bang's disease had never occurred in their certified herd; that a closed circuit existed between the milking machines and the milk bottles; and that the pipes through which the milk passed were sterilized daily with superheated steam. All workers were frequently examined for disease, and none suffering from an illness, regardless of how mild, was allowed to work in that department. The bacterial count of their certified milk averaged 2,500, whereas the law permitted 7,500. Therefore, it seemed safe to use raw certified milk.

The principal objection to giving raw milk to infants has been danger of undulant fever. The American Medical Association has recently stated that milk is probably never a carrier of this disease, which appears to come from handling meat of the diseased animals. When persons are violently opposed to giving unboiled, certified milk to an infant, I strongly suspect that they, like myself until recently, have not taken time to find out how superior it really is or how carefully it is produced. I feel that they may have lost sight of the fact that in trying to protect health, certain health protectors may be destroyed.

From the mother's point of view, the advantage of using certified milk is that it eliminates making a formula; you merely pour it into the nursing bottles. Nothing could be easier.

No raw milk other than certified is safe enough to be given to a baby. Even if you live on a farm and know your cows personally, so many bacteria gain access during milking that the milk should be boiled before being made into a formula.

Formulas of evaporated milk. Unless certified milk is available, evaporated milk is probably the best for a formula. The advantages of using evaporated milk are many: all brands are uniform in quality; the production of the milk to be canned is usually carefully supervised; the milk is homogenized; it is absolutely sterile; it is available everywhere and is easily stored; and it contains some added vitamin D. Any formula of evaporated milk can easily be made directly in the nursing bottles; measuring cups, mixing bowls, and other paraphernalia are not needed.

Kinds of milk not to use. There are many brands of milk on the market which should not be used. These are prepared particularly for infants' formulas and are said to "contain everything." They are sold in powdered form or in a liquid form similar to evaporated milk; only water need be added.

These milks supply some vitamins A, C, D, and the cheaper B vitamins but rarely in amounts adequate to produce optimum health. Certainly the needs of your individual baby are not taken into consideration. Such milks usually lack vitamins E, K, and P, several B vitamins, copper, iodine, unsaturated fatty acids, and other nutrients. Yet the assurance that these milks contain everything gives the mother a false sense of security and prevents her from making any attempt to improve her infant's diet.

The main disadvantage of such milk is the tremendous amounts of sugar it contains. One popular brand, for example, contains 56 per cent sugar. Babies fed such milk gain weight rapidly but are usually soft, pale, and flabby; they lack muscle tone and resistance to disease. They are frequently irritable, cry a great deal, and suffer from diarrhea and colic. They are the babies who cause mothers to worry themselves sick and to age a year for every month.

By giving your baby an inadequate formula, in all probability you will produce disease as surely and almost as quickly as a scientist produces disease in laboratory animals by placing them on diets high in refined sugar, low in protein, and deficient in other nutrients. Even though a sugar-loaded formula will cause an infant to gain weight rapidly, such a gain is not an indication of health. Rather it is like the gain of hogs fattened for market where only gain in weight is the object instead of health.

Unfortunately these prepared milks are widely used and are often recommended by seemingly well-trained pediatricians. In fact, in March, 1950, when I went to the hospital to pick up our tiny to-be-adopted daughter, the pediatrician in charge told me that she was to be given a formula of a preparation which I knew to contain 55 per cent sugar and which was deficient in perhaps a dozen essential nutrients. A quart of formula had been made up for me to take home. The prepared formula was, of course, "forgotten." I could not help thinking, however, of the many young mothers, perhaps frightened at their own inexperience and having little knowledge of nutrition, who would have followed such advice blindly. Yet each mother wants health for her baby just as much as I desired it for mine.

If such a milk is recommended to you, ask your pediatrician to allow you to make the formula of some other form of milk.

Formulas for premature infants. I frequently find that formulas of sugar-loaded prepared milks are being given to premature infants, the very babies who need the best formula possible. Mothers and all too often pediatricians are so eager for these tiny babies to gain that they lose sight of the fact that the smaller the baby, the greater is his need for protein and other nutrients which are far more essential than sugar. When a formula high in sugar is given in the mistaken belief that it is necessary to achieve a rapid gain in weight, normal growth may be sacrificed in favor of useless fat. Furthermore, the premature baby is less able to cope with colic, diarrhea, and other disturbances which may result from high-sugar formulas than is a full-term infant, whereas his mother is likewise in no condition to cope with a shrieking, colicky baby.

As has been repeatedly brought out in the studies cited earlier in this chapter, premature babies gain more rapidly and have fewer digestive upsets on formulas high in protein and fat but low in sugar than on sugar-loaded formulas. The limitations of sugar must be appreciated if a premature baby is to thrive. Since many of their mothers have suffered from toxemia (the major cause of premature births), these infants may be born deficient in choline and/or methionine (p. 55). The giving of yeast to supply choline and of undiluted milk to furnish ample methionine may be factors in saving the lives of these tiny infants.

What if my pediatrician does not agree? Formulas simulating breast milk have been recommended for decades and are still recommended by teachers in most medical schools. Medical journals have carried thousands of articles about standard formulas, whereas only a few articles have been published concerning the type of formula discussed in this chapter. Probably you will take your baby to the best doctor in town, who invariably is the most overworked pediatrician with too little time to read. Somehow he must keep up with the thousands of reports being published each month, not only on nutrition but also on endocrinology, antibiotics, the steroids, perhaps surgery, and a hundred and one other subjects. There is only one chance in a million that he may have read the articles cited in this chapter. Do not expect him to be familiar with them.

All physicians have seen dozens of "cures" and "improvements" come and go. In order to protect your baby's health, your pediatrician must be skeptical of any new approach until he has had time to investigate it. Furthermore, the field of nutrition has attracted more faddists and crackpots than almost any other field. If your physician is not skeptical when a formula he has never heard of is advocated by a person he has never heard of, then you had better take your baby to another pediatrician.

On the other hand, physicians are aware of the tremendous importance of protein, the need for fat, and the limitations of sugar. Few doctors, if any, would object to the formulas recommended in this chapter for the healthy infant. Babies, however, are individuals, and yours may present special problems which would call for a formula entirely different from those discussed here.

References are listed throughout this book for the use of your physician in case you wish to discuss any controversial point with him. In most cases, the studies cited have been conducted by professors in leading medical schools. These outstanding men are as eager for your baby to achieve health as are you and your own pediatrician.

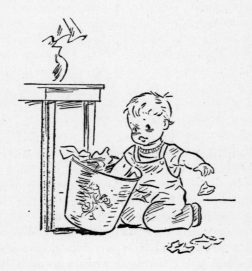

CHAPTER 12

FORMULAS ARE EASY TO MAKE

I ONCE heard a pediatrician remark, "Ninety per cent of all problems in baby feeding are mechanical." His statement may be true.

If the holes in the rubber nipple are too large, for example, or if the milk flow is too rapid for any reason, the baby is forced to gulp his food. Whenever he gulps, he swallows air. Bubbles of air form in his stomach and enlarge as they heat to body temperature; then they are burped up. If the air bubble is especially large, it comes up with such force that it may push before it what appears to be an entire bottle of formula. Much the same result occurs when the air inlet of the bottle is faulty. In this case, it is so difficult for the baby to get the milk that he must suck more and swallow more than if the milk flowed freely. With each swallow he forces air from his throat into his stomach where it eventually accumulates into large bubbles. Each time as the bubbles force their way up, he may lose much of his feeding.

How is an inexperienced mother to know that the cause is mechanical? Every time the baby is fed, he throws up. That must mean that he is sick or has a delicate stomach or that the formula does not agree with him. Probably she hurries to her pediatrician. Unless he happens to see her feeding the baby, he too has no way of knowing that faulty nipples or bottles are causing the difficulty. Perhaps, thinking that the formula is being poorly tolerated, he changes it. Since the same bottles are used, the new formula does not "agree" either. More worry; more time spent feeding the baby (an infant who has lost a meal will soon get hungry again); more energy used cleaning up after him; interrupted sleep at night. What to do now? Perhaps the mother takes the baby to another doctor who also changes the formula and possibly gives a sedative to "settle" the baby's stomach. The pattern may continue to repeat itself. Expenses mount and anxieties increase. Such can be the mechanical problems of baby feeding.

Since many such problems are caused by imperfect nursing bottles, the type of bottle you select can actually determine the degree to which you will enjoy your motherhood.

Selecting bottles. Probably the perfect nursing bottle is yet to be manufactured. In order to find what problems might occur, I have used nine different types of bottles. Some leak; some tip over easily; some have such faulty air inlets that the baby can get little milk; others allow the milk to flow so readily that the infant cannot satisfy his sucking instincts. The nipples of some can be removed so easily that, if you prop up the bottle, you may return to find your baby swimming in formula; other nipples are so tight that it is a major feat to get them on. The plastic bottles are so light that a 6-month-old baby can throw them at you; the nipples are so wobbly that it is almost impossible, without touching them with your hands, to force a toothpick through the holes if they become plugged. Since you have no way of knowing whether or not a bottle is satisfactory until you have used it and compared it with other bottles, my advice, especially to any mother whose baby throws up, is to buy one bottle each of several varieties. As bottles break, replace them with the ones you prefer. If I had done that when our son was tiny, it would have saved expense and endless energy.

I strongly recommend that you select bottles with mouths wide enough to put a spoon into them. Preparing the formulas directly in such bottles is the easiest and quickest method and eliminates sterilizing measuring cups, mixing bowls, and other paraphernalia.

Choose a type of bottle in which the nipple holes were made by the manufacturer; then try to leave the holes alone. Boiling the nipples causes the rubber to become softer, and the holes will enlarge quickly enough. If you feel you must burn in new holes, use the smallest needle sold. Even if your baby does not throw up after the holes are enlarged, the milk may flow so freely that he will be unable to satisfy his urge to suck; then unless a pacifier is given him, he will probably start sucking his thumb. Of the nine types of bottles I have used, the nipple holes made by the manufacturer are sufficiently large to permit the even flow of formulas containing yeast and some vegetable fibers. Instead of enlarging the holes, keep a box of hardwood toothpicks at your elbow as you feed the baby; if a hole becomes plugged, force a toothpick through it.

A good bottle must have air inlets which work efficiently. In order to appreciate how completely the milk flow is stopped when air does not enter the bottle as each sip of milk is withdrawn, try drinking a liquid from a narrow-necked bottle with your mouth over the top so that no air can enter. You will find that a vacuum or partial vacuum is created, and little or no liquid will flow into your mouth. Your baby, encountering the same situation, finds sucking so difficult that he may tire and stop eating when his hunger pangs are barely satisfied; he is soon hungry again. Such a baby not only throws up but wants to eat all the time.

This problem of air inlets caused me more grief than all other problems combined. The bottles I used at that time had been highly recommended. When our son would take only 2 or 3 ounces of formula at a feeding, even though other babies of his age were taking 8 or 9 ounces, we assumed that he was a dainty eater. In an hour or so, he wanted to eat again. Since he had to suck a great deal, he swallowed much air and threw up far more than he should. When other babies were sleeping throughout the night, our little imp was waking up the occupants of an entire apartment house with vigorous yells for food at least every 3 hours. Although my pediatrician assured me that the baby would outgrow such behavior, I had exactly one night of uninterrupted sleep during his first year. Since I used the same bottles in feeding our little girl, identical difficulties arose. Fortunately I decided to investigate different bottles and discovered what the trouble was.

Read the literature which comes with your bottles, and be sure you know where the air inlets are. The inlets of one popular brand are tiny holes in the base or flange of the nipples; mothers frequently do not know the holes exist. These holes become clogged easily, especially when yeast or vegetable water is used in the formula; they should be opened with a toothpick each time the nipples are washed.

I would not recommend narrow-necked bottles. They are difficult to clean. In using them, you must sterilize funnels, mixing bowls, measuring cups, and everything except the kitchen sink. It is uncanny how you can misplace the funnel and waste time hunting for it and using it, perhaps getting it too full and spilling the milk. My main objection is that such bottles sometimes interfere with good nutrition. There may be many times when your baby will howl with hunger; yet you have been too busy to prepare the formula in advance. If you are using wide-mouth bottles and giving an evaporated-milk formula, you can stir yeast, molasses, and vitamin C into the milk as the water heats; if you are using whole milk, you can pour it into the bottle, set the bottle in warm water, and then add the nutritional supplements. Most mothers I know who use narrow-necked bottles skip the supplements under such circumstances.

Do not take the claim of anticolic bottles seriously. Such a claim implies that the air an infant swallows comes from inside the bottle rather than from the mouth. These bottles are no more anticolic than is a human breast. I would not buy a bottle merely because it is heat resistant; all the bottles appear to be remarkably resistant to heat. Look for bottles with wide mouths, with holes already in the nipples, and with nipples which an older baby cannot remove. You can determine whether such a bottle is satisfactory in other respects only after you have used it.

When all goes well. As the baby nurses, there should be a steady stream of air bubbles going into the bottle. For most babies, these bubbles should be about ⅛ inch in diameter, allowing the infant to empty the bottle in approximately 20 minutes. When the bubbles are ¼ inch in diameter or larger, the baby is usually being forced to gulp air to such an extent that he may throw up, particularly if he is very young. Such bubbles indicate that the nipple holes are too big and/or that too much air is getting into the bottle. If the baby throws up or finishes the bottle in less than 20 minutes, buy new nipples and/or tighten the air inlets. If he continues to throw up, buy different bottles.

In case no bubbles can be seen, make sure the nipple holes are open. If they are and still no bubbles appear, the air inlet is faulty, and the baby is sucking against a vacuum. The air inlet is inefficient whenever air bubbles rush into the bottle as soon as it is taken from the baby's mouth; in this case, however, the nipple holes are too large. If the bubbles are tiny ($\frac{1}{16}$ inch in diameter or less), the baby is probably sucking against a partial vacuum. When the air inlet cannot be adjusted by loosening a screw-topped bottle or cleaning out air holes, it is usually best to buy a different kind of bottle, especially if your baby is only a few weeks old or if he takes 30 minutes or longer for a feeding.

Sterilizing equipment. Many young mothers have told me that they have become nervous wrecks by the time they have finished sterilizing the equipment and preparing the formula the first few times. There is no reason for getting yourself into a tizzy over such a problem. Sterilizing bottles and other paraphernalia is similar to steaming or boiling potatoes which you surely have done hundreds of times. You merely put the potatoes (bottles, spoons, tongs, etc.) in water, let them boil and take them out at a given time. You usually avoid handling hot potatoes; thus they remain sterile. Sterilizing bottles is as simple as that.

First scrub the bottles and nipples; test the nipple holes by forcing water through them; clean the air inlets; rinse thoroughly everything to be sterilized. If your pediatrician insists on a diffi-cult-to-prepare formula, sterilize the egg beater, mixing bowl, measuring cups, and all the other equipment you may need. Use a large pan with a sufficiently tight-fitting lid to hold the steam in; a deep well on your range is ideal. To prevent the bottles from breaking, place a rack in the pan; a small rack sold for roasting meat is satisfactory. In case you have no rack, use a folded tea towel. Provided the lid fits, 1 inch of water is sufficient; otherwise enough water should be used to cover everything to be sterilized.

Set the bottles, stirring spoons, tongs, and anything else you wish to sterilize in the water and cover the pan. As soon as the water begins to boil vigorously, check the time; allow 5 minutes for the bottles, and then put in the nipples and boil 1 minute longer. If you use a pressure cooker, bring the pressure to 5 pounds and boil the bottles 1 minute.

Rescue the tongs by the handle, and as soon as they are cool, remove the bottles and nipples, being careful not to touch anything which will come in contact with the baby's food or mouth. Instead of keeping the bottles on a tray, which takes up valuable work surface, prepare a sterile drawer as near the range as possible; scrub it and line it with boiled cloth which has been sundried or oven-dried; keep in the drawer any sterilized equipment you use for the baby. When a drawer is not available, keep the nipples in a sterile jar and leave the bottles in the sterilizing utensil until you use them.

Mothers are usually eager to know when they can stop sterilizing equipment. The time varies with the condition of your baby. If he has suffered digestive upsets, diarrhea, or some infection of the intestinal tract, you had better continue to sterilize his bottles and nipples until he is 1 year old or older. In case your baby has had no such upsets and is unusually healthy, you can probably stop when he is 6 months old. Ask your pediatrician to answer this question for you.

Making a formula. If you use raw certified milk, merely line up the sterile bottles and pour in the amount of milk the baby is accustomed to taking at each feeding. In case you are using supplements, add yeast, vitamin C, and blackstrap molasses; stir thoroughly or cap the bottles and shake them well before storing them in the refrigerator.

When pasteurized milk is given to an infant or when raw milk other than certified is used for a formula, boil the milk 3 minutes, cool it, and pass it through a sterilized strainer. The procedure is then the same as in making a formula of certified milk.

If you use evaporated milk, wash the can with soap and rinse it thoroughly before opening it. Some pediatricians recommend that the top be cleaned with cotton moistened with ethyl alcohol. For economy's sake, most of us like to make the amount of formula which will use a can, or 13 ounces, of milk. Line up the sterile bottles and pour in the boiling water. In case your formula is made of equal parts of water and milk, use only enough water to make half the amount of formula which the baby will usually take at a feeding. For example, if the baby customarily takes about 4 ounces of formula, line up six bottles and put slightly more than 2 ounces of water into each. Vitamin C and blackstrap molasses, if used, will dissolve more easily when added while the water is hot, but the evaporated milk (a little more than 2 ounces per bottle) should be added to cool the water before the yeast is stirred in.

In case you are using narrow-mouth bottles, mix the formula in a sterilized jar or measuring pitcher. Pour in the amount of water specified, add vitamin C and blackstrap, then the milk and lastly the yeast. Stir slightly, fill the bottles to the amount the infant will probably take at one feeding, cover them, and store them in the refrigerator.

Do not use distilled water in making a baby's formula. Ordinary water may be his only source of iodine and fluorine.

Adding vitamin C to a formula. If you wish to add vitamin C to a formula of certified or pasteurized milk, it is best to dissolve the tablets first. Drop 24 tablets, 100 milligrams each, into a small sterile jar, and pour ½ cup (24 teaspoons) of boiling water over them. Cover the jar and keep it in the refrigerator. By using these proportions, ½ teaspoon of the liquid will equal 50 milligrams of vitamin C. Shake the jar well each time before using. To each bottle of formula add ¼ teaspoon or more if you desire. Liquid vitamin-C preparations are available but are usually far more expensive and lower in potency than you yourself can prepare.

When an evaporated-milk formula is used, vitamin-C tablets can be put directly into the bottles; they will readily dissolve in hot water. Tablets of 50 milligrams each may be purchased; or 100-milligram tablets, which are usually cheaper, can be cut in half.

Since vitamin C which occurs naturally in foods is quickly destroyed by oxygen or heat, it is often feared that vitamin C added to a formula is not stable. The destruction of the vitamin in fresh foods is brought about by an enzyme, ascorbic acid oxidase, which is not present in the tablets. Studies have shown that synthetic vitamin C, added to a formula, loses little or none of its potency after being stored 4 days.

Adding blackstrap molasses and yeast to a formula. Despite its outstanding nutritive value, blackstrap molasses is so extremely laxative that no more than a few drops or at most ¼ teaspoon should be added to an entire day's formula at first. If the stools are not too soft, the amount can be increased gradually to as much as 3 teaspoons daily; larger amounts need not be used unless constipation is severe.

If you wish to use yeast, add no more than ¼ teaspoon to each bottle of formula for a newborn infant or for a baby of any age who has never been given yeast before. Increase the amount gradually, or by ¼ teaspoon every 3 to 5 days. Most month-old babies tolerate 1 level tablespoon of yeast daily; 6-month-old infants, 2 tablespoons. Larger amounts are probably not needed. Do not worry about lumps of yeast; if they do not disappear when the formula is stirred or shaken, they will settle to the bottom on standing.

In case you use a preparation of vitamins A and D in aqueous solution, add it and stir well before mixing in the yeast.

A special evening bottle may be valuable. It seems to me wise to make up a special stick-to-the-ribs evening bottle for the healthy baby who has had no colic or other digestive disturbances. Since cream, or fat, stays in the stomach longer than any other food, I advise putting 1 to 6 teaspoons more cream into this bottle than any other; it can be added, of course, only if you are using whole milk. Proteins also have a high stick-to-the-ribs quality; hence more brewers' yeast, which averages 46 per cent protein, can be put into this bottle. If you are using only 1 teaspoon of yeast daily, this entire amount might eventually go into the evening bottle. The daily quota of blackstrap molasses could also be put into this bottle and would identify it from other bottles. Since molasses stains clothing badly in case the baby burps up some of it, the stains are thus confined to the night clothes. You must, however, increase the amounts of cream, yeast, and molasses gradually; if all were increased at one time, the baby might suffer a digestive upset.

When the formula is made of evaporated milk and water, a more concentrated evening bottle could be prepared by using less water than in other bottles and/or by gradually adding more yeast and blackstrap.

Recently when I was talking with a pediatrician who donates a morning each week to a baby clinic, I spoke of my idea of an evening bottle, mentioning that mothers hesitated to use more evaporated milk than water in a formula. He laughed and told me that the formulas recommended for newborn infants as the mothers left our county hospital contained the proportion of 16 ounces of water to 8 ounces of evaporated milk. At least three times a month mothers bring to the clinic tiny infants who are thriving unusually well and gaining beautifully; invariably these mothers have become confused and are giving the babies formulas of 16 ounces of evaporated milk to 8 ounces of water. He stated that he does not bother to correct the mistake because the babies are thriving better on the concentrated formula than on the one recommended for them. Apparently you have little cause for worry if you add 1 or 2 extra ounces of evaporated milk to the evening bottle and withhold an equal amount of water.

In case you wish to introduce cereal, vegetables, or meat early, any or all of these foods might be put into the evening bottle (p. 146).

I have used a concentrated evening bottle in feeding our little girl and have recommended it to dozens of mothers. We all find that infants fed such a bottle sleep throughout the night at an earlier age than do most babies.

Vegetable water for formulas. When vegetables are boiled until tender and then allowed to soak, the cooking water contains appreciable amounts of iron, copper, potassium, magnesium, and other minerals; also the vitamins which readily dissolve in water but are not harmed by heat pass into the cooking water. Such water, therefore, can offer a valuable contribution when used in making an infant's formula. The water to be used may be that left from cooking the family's carrots, potatoes, or spinach, though usually there is not enough water from this source. I have found it more satisfactory to prepare special vegetable water.

I make formula water in a huge old coffee-pot because the spout is convenient and the pot does not take up much work surface; any utensil, however, would serve the purpose. Into this pot I put chopped parsley, celery, and carrot tops, trimmings from salad vegetables, tomato peelings if available, vegetables left on the dinner plates (they will be as sterile as surgical gauze after being boiled), and any clean trimmings available except those from the gas-forming vegetables of the cabbage family. Butchers often give away fresh parsley with each purchase of meat. If you can find a butcher who has a baby the same age as yours, he will probably give you parsley by the ton. Most grocers will allow you to take all the lettuce and celery trimmings you want. If you have a garden, save trimmings whenever you prepare vegetables and salad greens. Use tampala, chard, kohlrabi tops, and other vegetables not available in stores. Wash the vegetable trimmings, chop them slightly, pack them down in a utensil, and cover them with cold water; salt them lightly with iodized salt not only because it supplies iodine, sodium, and chlorine but also because salt draws juices out of the vegetables. Then boil slowly for 20 minutes or longer, and let the water and trimmings stand several hours or overnight. The more thoroughly the vegetables are cooked and the longer they stand, the larger are the amounts of nutrients which pass into the water. When you are ready to make the formula, reheat the vegetables and water to make sure the liquid is sterile; then pour it into the bottles through a small strainer covered with cheesecloth. Strain any remaining liquid into a jar and keep in the refrigerator. I usually try to make up enough for 3 or 4 days at a time.

If you do not have your own garden, there is always the problem of poison sprays which have been used on the vegetables. Perhaps they may more than counteract the value gained from such water at times; no one knows. If generous amounts of vitamin C are used in the formula, however, the poisons are apparently detoxified.

Although beet tops are undeniably nutritious, if you are an artistic soul, you had better avoid using them. The color of a formula made with them is revolting.

What formula did you use? Few women, I am sure, have been asked the question as often as I have, "What formula did you use?" Since babies are as much individuals as are adults, any formula must be adjusted to meet the problems of that particular infant. No formula, therefore, makes sense until you know a bit of the history of the baby for whom it was planned.

Our little boy, George, was 19 days old when we took him. He had previously been in a boarding home where he had received abominable care. He did not have a square millimeter of skin over his entire diaper region; blood even oozed from his buttocks. The folds of his neck were equally raw, and curds of soured milk lay deep among them. His head was covered with extremely thick "scalp cap." His bone development was poor: a tiny squeezed-together face with little space between the eyes; the frontal fontanel was so wide you could see the pulsations of his brain. His head was weak and wobbly, and his muscle tone was nonexistent. He did, however, have gorgeous blue eyes and infinite possibilities.

What this baby needed was food rich in protein and vitamins A and C to bring about the healing of his skin at all possible speed; and calcium and vitamin D to start his bones growing normally.

At that time I had not read of formulas without added sugar. His first formula contained 13 ounces of evaporated milk, 16 ounces of water, and 2 tablespoons each of milk sugar and yeast, the latter added for its protein content more than for B vitamins. I added no blackstrap molasses because I did not dare risk his having diarrhea. To accelerate healing, I put 100 milligrams of vitamin C into each bottle of formula. He was kept on a demand schedule. To supply vitamin D, I gave him 20 drops of cod-liver-oil concentrate daily, and until healing was complete, 20 drops of both halibut-liver oil and wheat-germ oil after each feeding.

Fortunately I knew a mother who was selling breast milk, and from her I was able to obtain enough milk to give the baby two or three feedings daily for 2 weeks. Another young mother came to the house and nursed him several times; still another, whose baby had been lost at birth, gave him some of her milk. His condition was such that his resistance to disease was probably nil; therefore I wanted most the antibodies supplied by breast milk.

It was a joy to see the child fill out and become healthy. Within 3 days his skin had completely healed; hence vitamin C was decreased to 300 milligrams for the day, and the halibut-liver oil and wheat-germ oil to 20 drops after one feeding. The only water ever used in his formulas was that in which vegetables had been cooked. Small amounts of blackstrap molasses were added from time to time, but it usually proved to be too laxative to be continued. After 2 weeks he was pronounced to be in excellent condition. Our pediatrician commented that the formula was rather concentrated but added that the infant was obviously thriving on it; he therefore saw no reason to change it.

I decreased the amount of sugar and increased the milk in the formula until, at 2 months, the baby was getting equal amounts of evaporated milk and vegetable water, 2 rounded tablespoons of yeast, ½ to 1 teaspoon of blackstrap molasses, 300 milligrams of vitamin C, and no added sugar. When the weather was hot, I added more water to the formula and used a bit more iodized salt in cooking the vegetables. If he was exposed to a cold or showed any signs of getting one, the amount of vitamin C in the formula was increased. In addition, he had orange juice almost daily. To supply additional vitamin P, I often chopped the white part of lemon rind and cooked it with the vegetables in making formula water. This same formula was used during the 22 months he drank from a bottle.

In contrast, our little girl, Barbara, was a beautiful specimen of babyhood. She was only 38 hours old when I took her from the hospital. She had amazing strength in her 8 pounds 3 ounces. Her bone structure was nearly ideal, her tiny dental arch perfect, her face wide and beautifully developed, and her tiny head as round as a golf ball and not pushed out of shape as the bones are when poorly calcified. The only count against her was that her natural mother had suffered from asthma since she herself was only 2 weeks old; the asthma had been continuous throughout her childhood and her pregnancy. The infant, therefore, was potentially allergic, and steps had to be taken in an attempt, at least, to prevent allergies from developing.

I have always mixed her formulas directly in the bottles. Her first formula, given when she was approximately 41 hours old, was 2 ounces each of evaporated milk and vegetable water; ½ teaspoon of yeast and a 100-milligram tablet of vitamin C were added to each bottle. The large amount of vitamin C was given because of the allergy history and because her umbilical cord was still healing. Not a grain of sugar, except that in blackstrap molasses, has ever been added to her milk. About ¼ to 1 teaspoon of molasses has been added to her evening formula whenever her stools were firm enough to allow it. Ten drops each of cod-liver-oil concentrate, halibut-liver oil, and wheat-germ oil were given her the day she came from the hospital, and all three oils were continued until she was 6 months old. I then decided to use the more easily absorbed preparations of vitamin A alone and vitamins A and D, both in aqueous solution. Two drops of each of the concentrates were added directly to the milk in every bottle of formula.

I gave her 3 ounces of fresh, undiluted orange juice as a source of vitamin P on her third day, and she has had 3 to 5 ounces daily since that time. The oranges, however, have been grown on soil rich in humus which, some persons claim, cause fewer allergies than do oranges grown with chemical fertilizers.

When Barbara was 2 weeks old, I attended a nutrition convention. There I talked to a number of physicians whose conviction it was that raw certified milk was superior to any other for infants' formulas. After that she was given certified milk rather than evaporated; the yeast, blackstrap, and vitamin C were added as before.

By the time she was 3 months old, she looked pale. Since she was not getting vegetable water, her diet was possibly deficient in iron. At my pediatrician's suggestion, I shook one capsule of powdered iron and copper * into her bottles daily and have continued giving her this supplement. In a short time she had the lovely high color that every baby should have.

This program is still continuing. The large amount of vitamin C is given with the full blessing of an allergy specialist aware of her prenatal history. We may be erring on the side of giving her too much, but since it is harmless, we believe that it is better to give too much than too little. To date she has shown no sign of allergy, and her progress has been satisfactory in every respect.

Since every infant has his own particular needs, the fact that I have used these formulas does not necessarily mean that they would be the best for your baby. They are, however, more adequate in the essential nutrients than are the usual formulas.

* Copperin B, produced by Myron L. Walker Co., Mount Vernon, New York.

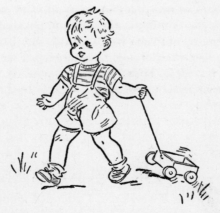

CHAPTER 13

START FROM BIRTH
TO PREVENT FEEDING PROBLEMS

CHILD-FEEDING problems as we know them today were almost nonexistent until about 30 years ago. Up to that time the problem more often was to prevent children from overeating. Instead of the familiar, "Drink your milk, Johnny," it was "Don't make a pig of yourself." During the last few decades, however, such problems have become so common that almost every mother going into a pediatrician's office complains that her child will not eat. This problem has many causes, among them the accumulation of hundreds of early frustrations associated with eating. Faulty technics used in the past few decades but not earlier have helped to produce this all-time high record of feeding problems.

The book which can help you more than any other to prevent such problems (and to enjoy your motherhood) is *The Rights of Infants* by Margaret Ribble (New York: Columbia University Press, 1943). The books most frequently recommended to mothers are *Infant and Child in the Culture of Today* by Arnold Gesell and Frances Ilg (New York: Harper and Brothers, 1943) and *Baby and Child Care* by Benjamin Spock (New York: Pocket Books, Inc., 1946). Both books are excellent. My feeling is, however, that if a mother thoroughly studies and applies Margaret Ribble's teachings, the problems so expertly discussed by Dr. Spock will not arise, and the child will progress along the normal lines so ably outlined by Dr. Gesell. In fact, I believe *The Rights of Infants* is so important that it should be required reading for all prospective mothers and for every medical student who expects to practice pediatrics.

Let us now see what faulty technics may have caused feeding problems to arise.

The 4-hour schedule. One technic which has undoubtedly contributed to feeding problems is the custom of keeping infants on a 4-hour schedule, totally disregarding the baby's individuality. Although many infants prefer to eat every 4 hours, by no means all of them do. If an infant wishes to eat at that interval, all goes well. What happens to the baby who is hungry at the end of 2 hours but is forced to wait until the clock says he may be fed again?

At first the infant frets, then cries, and is soon screaming; the screaming may continue for an hour or more. The household is upset by the noise; the father probably becomes irritable; by feeding time the mother is such a nervous wreck that, if she is nursing the baby, her anxiety has probably retarded her milk flow. In any case, the infant has gulped so much air during his screaming that he may feel full; perhaps he has so exhausted himself that when he is allowed to eat, he can probably take little food. Because of the air swallowed, he may throw up much of his food as the air bubbles escape. Some of the swallowed air may have passed into his intestines where it continues to heat to body temperature and to expand, resulting in gas pains and colic. The vomiting and colic cause the mother and perhaps the physician to conclude that the breast milk or formula does not agree with the infant; he may be taken from the breast or changed from one formula to another.

Since the baby is too exhausted to eat much, he may soon doze off to sleep. The mother usually feels that he must nurse more or take a certain amount of formula; hence she goes through a process of pinching his cheek, patting his feet, and moving him from one position to another in an attempt to force him to eat. Perhaps she succeeds to the extent of another ½ ounce.

If the child has eaten little or has thrown up, he will certainly want to eat again before another 4-hour period has elapsed. Yet such liberty is not to be tolerated. The screaming and entire barbaric procedure may be repeated. Despite the fact that evidence now exists that the 4-hour schedule is often harmful to both mother and child, such schedules have by no means been completely discarded.

How do *you* like to wait for food: those late Thanksgiving and Christmas dinners when you starve for hours before being allowed to eat? How would you like to be awakened and forced to eat? Let us suppose you have eaten all you want and have fallen into a restful sleep. Your husband, let us say, pats your feet, pinches your cheek, turns you gently from side to side, and starts shoving food into your mouth. As you awake, you would probably exclaim, "What in heaven's name are you trying to do?" He might answer, "I don't think you ate enough before going to sleep." If you doze off again and the procedure is repeated, not once but four or five times daily, you will conclude that you had married the wrong man and will probably divorce him. Yet this technic is still being used daily on thousands of infants. Certainly it causes unpleasant associations with eating which can carry over into feeding problems later.

The demand schedule. It is important to realize that the infant has no conception of time; he knows only his own rhythms. The demand schedule recognizes these rhythms, and when it is followed, the infant is allowed to eat whenever he chooses and the amount he chooses. Actually most babies soon put themselves on a schedule which is often so regular that you can set a clock by it. The demand schedule has been studied thoroughly [1,2,3] and has been found not only to result in happier, more secure infants and more relaxed mothers but also to help prevent feeding problems.

The late Dr. Aldrich, when in the Pediatrics Department at the Mayo Clinic, made a study of 668 infants whose mothers were told to feed them whenever they were hungry and to allow them

[1] C. A. Aldrich and E. S. Hewitt, "A Self-regulating Feeding Program for Infants," *J. Am. Med. Assn.*, 135 (1947), 340.

[2] C. K. Rowan-Legg, "Self-Demand Feeding of Infants," *Canadian Medical Association Journal*, 60 (1949), 388.

[3] K. Glaser, "Self-Demand Feeding Schedule," *Am. J. Dis. Child.*, 75 (1948), 309.

to take any amount of food they preferred. Of 100 of these babies, only 2 were eating irregularly when 1 month old; 10 were eating every 2 hours; 62 every 3 hours; and only 26 every 4 hours. At 2 months, half of the babies were eating every 3 hours and half every 4 hours. By 3 months, most of them had put themselves on a 4-hour schedule. Although other records have been similar, this study alone shows that few infants can tolerate a 4-hour schedule from birth without frustration associated with eating.

Many articles now appearing in the *Journal of Pediatrics* and similar magazines stress that no physician should specify the amount of formula a baby should take at any feeding. They advise allowing the baby to eat only as much as he wants, regardless of how little or how much.

Dr. Aldrich also made a study of the causes and frequency of crying among newborn infants while in the hospital and after being taken home. Crying was recorded as such only when a period of screaming lasted for 3 minutes or longer. The infants were fed every 3 hours while in the hospital. The mothers were instructed to keep them on demand schedules at home and to use "such soothing devices as a rocking chair and lullabies." (What a refreshing statement to read in a medical journal!) It was found that the main cause of crying at this age was hunger. While in the hospital, the infants averaged eleven crying spells per day, certainly an argument for taking them home as quickly as possible. During the first week at home the average was four crying spells.

If any of us experienced intense unhappiness associated with food even four times daily, we would soon come to think of eating as an unpleasant affair. When a baby is given a pacifier to suck while the bottle heats or a mother gets ready to nurse him, crying from hunger can be largely eliminated, and with it this particular frustration associated with food.

All studies made of demand schedules report that mothers are tremendously relieved to know the restrictions are lifted; that the babies are happier and more contented, and as they grow older, cry little if at all. One of the surprising findings is that by the time the infants are 3 or 4 months old, they develop amazing patience in waiting to be fed. Apparently they are already secure in knowing that hunger is followed by food, not by frustration. In growth and general development, babies kept on demand schedules have been found to be equal or superior to infants fed every 4 hours.

Buy a rocking chair. In my opinion the most important piece of furniture to obtain when preparing for a baby is a good rocking chair, preferably a platform rocker with strong high arms and a high back on which a tired mother can comfortably rest her head. Although it may seem far fetched, a rocking chair is important in preventing feeding problems.

It is assumed that, during the last months of pregnancy when the infant's nervous system has become fairly well developed, the protection of the uterus gives the unborn baby a feeling of the greatest possible security. Every time the mother moves, whether walking or turning in bed, her baby is gently rocked. If possible, this same feeling of security should be given the infant after birth and should be associated with eating.

It is now conceded that an infant who has been nursed becomes a better adjusted child and adult because he has been held, loved, protected, and made to feel secure while he has been fed. An infant who associates pleasure with eating rarely develops feeding problems later. The same association of pleasure and food can be given to a bottle-fed baby provided the mother holds him.

Few mothers, however, will consistently hold a baby during his feedings unless they enjoy doing so. When the mother does not have a comfortable rocking chair, she may feel too tired to hold him and may resort to propping up his bottle. After the baby is 4 or 5 months old, he becomes heavy to hold; the mother will be even more inclined to prop up the bottle if she has no chair with strong supporting arms.

When the bottle is propped up, the feeding may go well and the infant will lack only the feeling of love and security he would receive if he had been held. On the other hand, many frustrations may result: the bottle may move out of the infant's reach; the nipple holes may become plugged up; the air inlet may be faulty, and the child must suck against a vacuum; or the nipple may mash together or turn inside out because of the vacuum. Since it is difficult to swallow when lying down, the infant whose bottle is propped up is forced to gulp large amounts of air; hence he may associate stomach discomfort and perhaps vomiting and choking with eating. Such frustrations, which could be largely avoided if the mother held her baby, may contribute later to feeding problems.

I do not wish to imply that under no circumstances should the bottle be propped up, but that such times should be held to a minimum. Probably every mother finds that at times her attention must be given to other members of the family. Also there may be times when a bottle holder serves a valuable purpose (p. 87). As the infant grows older and is loved and played with by all members of the family, his need to be held during feeding somewhat diminishes. Whenever a bottle is propped up, however, the mother should glance at her baby frequently to see that all is going well.

Early baby feeding. In the days when feeding problems rarely existed, babies were given no solid foods until they were about 1 year old, except an occasional nibble from the family table. The current practice of introducing foods extremely early almost always results in feeding problems. Nature protects the tiny infant by prompting him to force semisolid substances from his mouth. Even with utmost care and patience, it is almost impossible to prevent a young infant from associating displeasure with eating when a basic instinct is ignored. Furthermore, his control over his tongue is so immature and his tiny throat muscles are so underdeveloped that he cannot swallow solid foods easily.

Have you ever watched a mother, perhaps too tired or too busy to be patient, carry out instructions to feed her 4- or 6-week-old infant 1 or 2 tablespoons of cereal? The baby is held in a half-reclining position while the mother stuffs food into his mouth. He immediately forces it out. She scrapes the messy cereal from his chin and jabs it back into his mouth. This horrible procedure of stuffing in and forcing out may go on for ½ hour or more before the specified amount of cereal has disappeared. In my opinion this atrocious violation of nature can be the beginning of the most serious feeding problems later.

It is possible to give an adequate diet without solid foods. Studies have been made in the Pediatrics Departments of Johns Hopkins University [4] and Cornell University Medical School [5] in which infants were given formulas fortified with vitamins and minerals and were fed no food except cereal until they were 9 months old. The cereal was introduced at 6 months and then only in the quantity the infants wished to take. The babies were examined every 2 weeks, x-rays were taken of their bones, and biochemical analysis was made of blood and excreta. Their development was compared with that of other infants fed solid foods early. The babies in each group were found to be equally healthy.

If solids must be introduced before your baby is 3 or 4 months old, dilute them with milk or fruit juice and give them from a bottle. This method saves the mother time and rarely antagonizes the baby. Use a hatpin to burn large holes in the nipple, or cut a hole in it. A still better procedure is to force a hardwood toothpick into each hole and leave them there while you boil the nipple; when the toothpicks are removed the resulting holes are smooth rather than jagged as they are when cut or burned.

Dr. Rowan-Legg, Dr. Aldrich, and many other physicians, writing for their fellow pediatricians, stress that solid foods should not be introduced to all babies at a certain age and that quantity should not be specified; that babies vary so widely in their ability to swallow, one infant may be ready for solids months before another; and that one baby will enjoy eating perhaps 2 tablespoons of food, whereas another of the same age may revolt at a bite. The infant's individuality must be considered if he is to

[4] E. V. McCollum and W. Grubb, "A Completely Supplemented Evaporated Milk and Its Use as a Food for Infants," *Am. J. Dis. Child.*, 68 (1944), 231.

[5] A. J. Vignec, H. McNamara, and H. L. Barnett, "Use of a Supplemented Milk for Infant Feeding," *Am. J. Dis. Child.*, 76 (1948), 154.

enjoy his food. Let him decide when he wants to begin solids, and let him eat as much or as little as he desires.

Taking away the bottle. During the period when feeding problems have become almost the rule rather than the exception, it has been customary to take the bottle away from a baby when he was 6 to 9 months old, regardless of how desperately he may still want it. Many such infants have gone on hunger strikes when offered milk from a cup. The result has often been weeks of unhappiness and frustration for both the baby and the mother, one stormy session following another. Many mothers have spent hours spooning milk into their children who have been antagonized to the extent that they refuse to drink from a cup. Aside from associating unpleasantness with food in general, infants weaned too early, particularly if weaned against their will, tend to become non-milk drinkers later.

Avoid having your baby associate this frustration with eating; allow him to drink from a bottle as long as he wishes, regardless of what your neighbors think. You can be quite sure he will not take his nursing bottles to college with him.

Good feeding habits have been produced. Dr. Aldrich and Dr. Hewitt (ref. 1, p. 142) set out to see whether feeding problems could be prevented. In their study of 668 babies, they told the mothers to offer food from time to time but to start feeding solids only when the babies seemed eager to eat and were able to swallow easily. Even then the foods were to be given in the amounts the babies desired, and no food which a baby rejected was to be forced upon him. Spoons and cups were to be used only when little hands reached for them. The mothers were advised to continue giving bottles until the babies themselves rejected them.

A few of these babies ate three meals daily as early as the fourth month, but the majority did not put themselves on regular meals until they were 9 months old. Most of the babies were still drinking milk from the bottle when they were 1 year old, at which time the study was terminated.

At the end of this study, the mothers were asked if their babies had ferocious appetites, if they sometimes needed to be coaxed to eat, or if they ever refused food or vomited. Most of the mothers (86 per cent) felt that their children had unusually good appetites, whereas 6 per cent reported the appetites to be huge. Of the entire group, less than 1 per cent of the mothers felt that their children ate too little. Feeding problems at this period at least had been almost completely avoided.

Once again the wisdom of our grandmothers is verified by scientific research. If you use these procedures recommended both by our grandmothers and by the Pediatrics Department of the Mayo Clinic, the chances are you, too, will avoid many feeding problems.

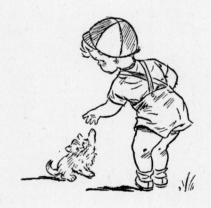

CHAPTER 14

CONTROVERSIES
APPLYING TO ALL BABIES

IT SEEMS to me that every detail concerning infant care and feeding is controversial. You can get yourself—if you have not already—into red-hot arguments over such questions as how frequently to change diapers, whether or not to add sugar to a formula, the comparative merits of 4-hour versus demand schedules, and a hundred and one similar problems. To argue logically about pacifiers is as impossible as to discuss religion or politics sanely.

The subjects in this chapter are particularly controversial. I am not at all sure I have the right answers. Please disagree with my points of view as heartily as you wish. Together, however, we may arrive at worth-while conclusions.

Can spitting up be prevented? Spitting up milk is almost as universal as babyhood and is usually accepted as inevitable. Yet it adds greatly to the work, and sometimes worry, of a mother and certainly detracts from the appeal of the baby. We have all seen babies who, if sprinkled with dill sauce, would smell like a delicatessen most of the time even though their mothers were continually bathing them and changing their clothing. With our first baby, I thought that spitting up was a rather unforgivable act of nature. I have now concluded that, in my case at least, it results only from poor mothering. I strongly believe that most spitting up can be prevented, although I know of several uncooperative infants, beautifully mothered, who seem bent on ruining my theory. Let us see what actually causes spitting up.

Many people, including some physicians, say that an infant

spits up merely because he overeats. If this argument were true, one could feed the baby more frequently or make the food more concentrated so he would have no desire to overeat; then the problem would be solved.

Almost everyone will agree that swallowed air is the principal cause of spitting up. In fact, air bubbles can be seen in x-rays of infants' stomachs. As the air heats to body temperature, it expands, and the bubble becomes larger; it may be expelled with such force that it pushes up any milk which happens to lie above it. The problem, therefore, becomes one of trying to keep the baby from swallowing excessive amounts of air and/or of burping him before large air bubbles can form.

If the baby usually spits up after nursing for 6 minutes or after taking 4 ounces of formula, try burping him after you have nursed him 3 minutes or after he has taken only 2 ounces of formula. A persistent "spitter-upper" should be burped even more frequently. It is often wise to burp a baby not only in the middle of each feeding and immediately after he has finished eating, but also 15 minutes to ½ hour later. Air swallowed at the end of the meal can remain in the stomach and not be heated sufficiently to form a large bubble until an interval of time has passed. If the infant is not burped again, he may throw up in spite of your feeling that you burped him thoroughly.

There are many reasons why babies swallow more air than they should. One of the commonest causes is that the infant may be allowed to remain in a reclining position while he eats. Just to see how difficult it is, every mother should try drinking a liquid while she is lying down. If you watch an adult taking refreshments as he reclines on a back prop at the beach or on a chaise longue in a cool patio, he will invariably lean forward each time he takes a sip. It is much easier to swallow with gravity as an aid.

If you hold a baby in a reclining position when you feed him or if you leave him in his crib and prop up the bottle or nurse him while you are lying down, his difficult swallowing causes him to use so much force that he cannot avoid pushing large amounts of air into his stomach. Unless the infant is burped frequently, you can expect him to spit up. A good rule to follow is to hold the baby in as nearly a <u>sitting position</u> as possible while you feed him; thus you can make sure that the esophagus is perpendicular and that gravity can aid in the swallowing. One mother told me that she had always followed this rule, and that her three children had never once spit up.

The infant who gulps his foods forces much air into his stomach and usually spits up badly. Sometimes a mother's milk flows so freely that all a baby can do is to gulp it. In this case, the baby must be burped more frequently than most infants. If the baby is bottle fed, perhaps the nipple holes are too large (p. 126) or the nipples are so old that the holes stretch easily. The obvious remedy is to buy new nipples.

Whenever an infant is overhungry, he wolfs his milk; perhaps he has been allowed to sleep too long between feedings or is kept on a 4-hour schedule rather than on a demand schedule. Probably the main reason why spitting up is taken for granted is that during these last decades, when 4-hour schedules were in vogue, the vast majority of tiny infants have been made to wait until they were almost starved before they were fed. As a result they gulped both food and air, and spitting up became the rule rather than the exception. The few infants who did not spit up were probably the rare ones who preferred a 4-hour schedule or were too weak to suck vigorously.

Many times a formula is so diluted that a baby is starved by the time he wakes up, even though he is on a demand schedule. I recently had a letter from a worried mother of a 5-month-old baby, complaining that he spit up far too much. She was giving him a formula of 13 ounces of evaporated milk, 24 ounces of water, and 6 tablespoons of sugar. The large amount of sugar readily satisfied his appetite, but there was little fat or protein to stick to his ribs and to give him sustained satiety. Naturally he wolfed his food and spit up.

A strong, vigorous baby often spits up more than does a weak one, simply because he can suck faster whenever he is hungry and therefore gulps more air. Many times an infant will spit up infrequently if at all when he is young; as he grows older and stronger, he may spit up a great deal. The solution in such a case is to make sure he is fed before he becomes overhungry and then to burp him frequently during each feeding. On the other hand, a baby with strong muscle tone often throws up little because he can easily contract the muscles of his stomach and abdomen and force up air bubbles while they are still small.

The infant who spits up a great deal naturally loses the nutritive value of some of his food and in time may become less healthy. For this reason alone spitting up should be prevented whenever possible.

If each of the suggestions given here is followed, I believe you will find that spitting up can be largely eliminated, your work decreased, and your motherhood made more pleasant.

Can thumb sucking be prevented? Thumb sucking in infancy appears to be a normal activity. Almost every obstetrician has seen babies suck their thumbs before they are off the delivery table. A few will tell you of an occasional infant who has sucked his thumb as soon as his head and one arm was delivered. It may be that all healthy fetuses suck their thumbs as a preparation for obtaining food after birth. We will agree, however, that thumb sucking as a habit—continued perhaps until the child is 5 or 6 years old—should be prevented if possible.

Psychologists tell us that sucking is a primary instinct which must be satisfied before the baby can be happy and well adjusted. Moreover sucking helps a newborn infant to breathe by aiding the movements of the diaphragm and by opening the air sacs in his lungs.

It is said that ample sucking during the first few months helps to develop muscles to be used in talking; and that if sufficient sucking is not allowed, speech difficulties may occur later. During these past 30 years, when 4-hour schedules were adhered to, babies were given little opportunity to suck. Interference with this basic instinct is thought to be largely responsible for the fact that hundreds of thousands of children now have speech difficulties and almost every large school must have its speech-correction teachers. Many such children, invariably nervous and high-strung, have been referred to me. They are not stutterers, although many have hesitancies in their speech. The ones I have seen were alert and intelligent youngsters, badly frustrated because they simply cannot talk so that anyone, except perhaps their parents, can understand them.

I have made a point of asking the mothers about the sucking satisfaction of their babies during infancy. Without exception I have been told pathetic stories of infants kept on 4-hour schedules, of bottles being taken away as early as the fifth month, and of thumb sucking being prevented by steel thimbles, arm braces, and other mechanical means. One mother told me her baby had never been taught to drink from a bottle and persistently refused one when her milk dried up, although he was only 4 months old. Another told of her baby's devotion to one particular nipple, and when it wore out, he refused all other kinds. Always came the tragic remark, "If I'd only known sucking was important!"

Dorothy Baruch, in her *Newer Ways of Discipline,* points out that ample sucking during infancy prevents thumb sucking later. If the sucking instinct is ungratified, the child sucks his thumb until he is perhaps 5 or 6 years old or older; the unsatisfied sucking instinct may then take the form of incessant gum chewing. Still later, if the child is a boy, he may spend much of his adult life sucking the stem of a pipe. How such assertions are proved I have no idea, but I certainly cannot disprove them. Can you?

The general acceptance of the demand schedule is a tremendous step in the prevention of thumb sucking. In addition, much sucking satisfaction is gained if the mother can allow her baby to remain at her breast as long as he desires. Often an infant will suck gently for 20 minutes or longer after he has withdrawn all the milk he will take. Similarly, if a bottle-fed baby is held until he has satisfied his appetite, is burped, and then put to bed with the bottle (still containing 1 or 2 ounces of milk) propped up, he may still suck for a long time, withdrawing little or no milk. Another means of preventing thumb sucking is to keep the nipple holes so small throughout the entire first year that the infant must work for every mouthful of food he gets. Discard old nipples as soon as the milk flows freely. Also keep the air inlets tight enough to make the infant of even 8 or 10 months take at least 20 minutes for each feeding.

Even when sucking opportunities seem ample, an unhappy or poorly mothered infant may suck his thumb as a comfort mechanism. Such sucking frequently results when the mother is too busy with other small children to rock her baby, cuddle him, sing him lullabies, and otherwise mother him as she would like to do. The remedy in this case is obvious, although sometimes impossible.

The seriousness of an unsatisfied sucking instinct goes beyond mere thumb sucking. As Pavlov first showed in dogs and as it has been proved repeatedly in humans, unhappiness and frustration can drastically interfere with the normal digestion and absorption of foods. Regardless of how adequate the diet, frustration may eventually cause serious malnutrition. The frustration of an infant resulting from being denied sufficient opportunity to suck very probably plays a causative role in the onset of allergies and other psychosomatic diseases.

If, after you have given your baby every opportunity to suck and have mothered him the best you can, he still sucks his thumb, by all means let him do so. It was formerly believed that thumb sucking caused malformed jaws and crooked teeth. Numerous studies have shown that if thumb sucking is given up before the permanent teeth erupt, as it usually is, little harm is done. Furthermore, many children who suck their thumbs persistently but whose diets are adequate in the bone-forming nutrients still have well-formed dental arches and straight teeth.

Are pacifiers justified? In case you have never seen a pacifier, it is a rubber nipple fastened to a plastic disk and ring. Its purpose is to give a baby something to suck. Our grandmothers and their grandmothers used them, chiefly to keep their babies quiet. As our civilization became germ conscious, pacifiers dropped into disgrace as being filthy and bacteria laden. However, now that sucking is recognized as a primary instinct which, if not fulfilled, can lead to severe emotional maladjustment, pacifiers are back in style.

Four years ago I watched a young mother nurse her month-old baby. Her milk flowed so freely that it fairly poured into the infant's mouth; if he had sucked strongly, he might have been drowned. The mother was worried because he sucked his thumb persistently. I offered to buy pacifiers for her, and although I must have gone into a dozen drugstores, the clerks gave me only puzzled stares and brought teething rings to show me. In contrast, I asked a druggist for pacifiers last week.

"We simply can't keep them in stock," he replied. "Every physician in town is recommending them."

Some people argue that pacifiers should not be used because infants get into the habit of sucking and therefore suck their thumbs whenever the pacifier is taken away. Experiments have shown exactly the opposite to be true. For example, a study was made of babies fed on exactly the same schedules and treated identically except that half of them were allowed to suck pacifiers as much as they liked. The pacifiers were first given to the babies when they were 2 days old. Despite the fact that these infants were in a foundling home where one would expect them all to suck their thumbs because of lack of mothering, not one infant given a pacifier sucked his thumb, whereas most of the other infants did.

The criticism that pacifiers are dirty is undoubtedly valid in some cases. Thumbs are often dirty, too. Although pacifiers cannot be boiled, they can be thoroughly sterilized by being soaked in soap suds or in alcohol. The next time you serve Martinis, you might drop in pacifiers instead of the olives.

Another argument against pacifiers is that they cause the babies to swallow air. I have not found this to be true nor have any mothers I know who have used them. Since there is no hole in the nipple and no liquid for the infant to swallow, I doubt that this form of sucking increases air swallowing.

The usual criticism of pacifiers is that they "look so terrible"—scarcely a valid argument against anything which is for the best welfare of your baby. I personally think they look cute wobbling from nose to chin, principally because the infants I have seen with pacifiers have been utterly relaxed, happy, and contented.

In my opinion, pacifiers are worth their weight in gold in keeping peace in the household. Often a young infant will scream lustily several times during the night. The adults in the house, who may need sleep badly, are repeatedly awakened and perhaps cannot go back to sleep readily. The result is general irritability and perhaps family quarrels the following day. When a pacifier is used, all is silent while the mother prepares to nurse her baby or heats his bottle. The same is true of the period before dinner when the older children and husband are hungry, tired, and perhaps irritable, and meal preparation demands your full attention. It is uncanny how an infant will select this time to add to the noise of radio or television by being fretful. Again, a pacifier saves the day. Every mother I know who has used one agrees with me.

If you wish to use pacifiers, introduce them as early as possible, preferably when the infant is less than 1 week old. The younger the baby, the greater is his need for sucking. Furthermore, an older baby will often refuse the pacifier, especially if first offered one when he is hungry. In case you have no pacifiers on hand, any nipple stuffed firmly with cotton can serve as a substitute. Many mothers, disliking a pacifier, wait until an infant starts to suck his thumb in earnest, then become alarmed, and belatedly try to force the baby to suck one, invariably without success.

Tiny infants will usually hold on to a pacifier like grim death, but a 3- or 4-month-old baby will often lose his pacifier and be unable to recover it. A trick which my neighbors and I have found most successful is to remove the ring from a pacifier, fasten the disk and nipple into a screw-topped nursing bottle, and place the bottle in the bottle holder. Then the baby can return to it as he wishes.

Many mothers ask me how long a baby may want to use a pacifier. Most babies, if allowed to suck all they wish, appear to have satisfied their sucking instincts and will give up a pacifier of their own accord by the time they are 4 or 5 months old. The time varies with the amount of other sucking they are allowed. If they are kept on demand schedules and the nipple holes are small enough to restrict the sucking time per bottle to at least 20 minutes, the pacifier is soon given up.

If you dislike pacifiers, however, thumb sucking certainly has been, and can be, prevented without them.

Does a baby need drinking water? A neighbor of mine dropped in the other day. In the course of our conversation she chanced to say, "I'm eternally fighting with Chucky to get him to drink water. He just won't drink enough."

"I'm always trying to talk Geordie out of wanting to drink it," I replied. She looked at me in surprise. "When he asks for a drink," I explained, "I usually say, 'How about a glass of milk?' and as a rule he settles for that. If he says no, then I suggest one juice after another, starting with orange juice as the most nutritious and working down the line. If he still persists, though he rarely does, he can have all the water he wants."

The reason for my attitude is that any beverage is mostly water; whole milk is 88 per cent water, most fruit juices about 90 per cent, tomato juice about 95 per cent. When a child drinks milk, he obtains protein, vitamins A and B$_2$, calcium, and other nutrients; if he selects juice, he probably gets vitamin C and several minerals. From either milk or juice he gets natural sugar, important in maintaining a cheerful between-meals disposition. In every case, he gets water.

A 10-pound baby will probably drink about 1 quart of milk a day and a few ounces of orange juice, provided he is healthy and allowed to have as much as he wants. For a baby 1 quart of liquid is roughly equivalent to 13 quarts daily for a 130-pound woman. Certainly that amount should be adequate.

There are several reasons why giving much water may not be a good idea. In the first place, it can satisfy the appetite temporarily and thus crowd out more nutritious foods. Second, there are many nutrients which readily dissolve in water: vitamins C and P, all the B vitamins, iodine, salt, and several minerals.

When much water is drunk, large quantities of these nutrients can be washed out of the body and lost in the urine. Experimental animals are readily killed by being forced to drink too much water; their deaths are caused by the loss of salt. Similarly deficiencies of the B vitamins have been produced by the same method even though the diet was adequate.

On especially hot days, any infant should be given an extra amount of water, but it seems to me easier for the mothers and the babies when the water is merely added to the formula for that day. Larger amounts of juice can also be given. In case a baby is kept on a 4-hour schedule, however, and is not allowed a pacifier, the giving of drinking water then becomes extremely important as a means of allowing him to fulfill his need for sucking, let nutritional losses be what they may.

Our little girl has never tasted water as such. Our boy had his first drink of water when he watched a gardener drink from a hose and tried it himself. Yet my attitude may be wrong. At least I was once firmly put in my place by a woman who listened to my views and then fairly snorted, "Well, when I'm thirsty, nothing tastes so good as a big glass of cold water." We will all agree, but one is rarely thirsty after drinking a glass or two of milk or fruit juice.

Is crying necessary for health? I cannot help questioning the old belief that crying develops an infant's lungs and should be allowed as a desirable "exercise." The infant's first cry on the delivery table is undeniably important; crying during the first 3 or 4 days may also help in opening the air sacs in the lungs. Crying after the age of 2 weeks, however, if purposely tolerated in the name of health, seems to me either an excuse for poor mothering or an acceptance of a faulty situation which one has no intention of remedying.

I recently dropped in on a friend to see her 6-week-old daughter. The infant was screaming her head off; yet the mother was going placidly about her work.

"This is her crying time," the mother explained cheerfully. "We always let her cry at this time. It's good exercise for her."

I hope this case is an isolated one, but I doubt it. Many mothers of well-fed infants have told me that they worried because their babies did not cry enough "to exercise their lungs."

Frequent, hard crying on the part of an infant can seriously interfere with his general nutrition. In all probability, the flow of digestive juices and the production of digestive enzymes are inhibited by his crying. It is conceivable that hard crying might easily interfere with the adequate absorption of food.

A healthy baby, who is kept on a completely adequate diet, who is loved and well mothered and whose needs are fulfilled, may go for days and even weeks without crying. He will fret when he is hungry or has a bubble pressing against his stomach or perhaps has soiled diapers, but little more. The assumption that all babies cry a great deal is probably based on the fact that most babies always have. Until about 1920, infants were usually well mothered, but their diets were often so deficient in the B vitamins and vitamins C and D that the wonder was they ever stopped crying. During the past 30 years, which could aptly be called the infants' Dark Ages, babies were made to wait for their food, were not allowed to suck as much as they liked, were not picked up when they wanted to be, and were not cuddled and loved as they should have been; certainly they had every right to cry, and they did. Furthermore, their diets could scarcely be considered adequate. Unfortunately the Dark Ages of babyhood are not yet over.

I strongly suspect that allowing an infant to scream in the name of "good exercise" or even to cry frequently without being comforted is in part responsible for the tremendous increase in allergies and other psychosomatic diseases during these past decades. A baby probably feels no more refreshed by crying than would you or I. Eventually the time may come when the infant who is usually quiet except for his laughter and vocalizing will be looked upon as one who is well nourished and well mothered.

Can oiling a baby be harmful? A problem which has worried me for many years is that of the use of baby oils. Most of the baby oils on the market are mineral oil. Not infrequently one meets a mother who rubs oil on her infant daily.

It is known that oil, rubbed on the skin, can be absorbed into the body. It is also known that mineral oil taken internally is not digested; yet some 40 per cent has been found to pass into the blood, where it is carried throughout the body. Provitamin A, or carotene, and vitamins A, D, E, and K dissolve in oil just as sugar dissolves in water. Thus mineral oil has been found to absorb these vitamins from the food mass in the intestines, from the cells of the intestinal walls, and from the blood itself. Eventually the oil, laden with these vitamins, passes into the large intestine to be excreted.

A mother recently consulted me about her two little girls. She was an intelligent woman, seemingly a most conscientious mother, well informed in nutrition. Yet the children were anything but healthy. They had had one cold after another and sieges of bronchitis and pneumonia; one child had suffered a middle-ear infection. Both children had had a series of sties, and one was just recovering from pink eye. The pores of the skin on their upper arms, knees, and buttocks were plugged with dead cells indicating, as did their history of infections, severe deficiencies of vitamin A. Their faulty bone structure showed an equally dire lack of vitamin D.

I asked the mother question after question. The diet she gave her children seemed to be adequate in every respect. I was completely baffled. Quite by chance, in telling me how dry the children's skin was, she mentioned that she had to rub them with baby oil several times daily, using a pint of oil each week. The brand she used I knew to be mineral oil. Could it be that the oil, absorbing through the skin, was robbing the children's bodies of vitamins A and D?

A few years ago *The Journal of the American Medical Association* carried an editorial pleading with physicians to stop recommending the internal use of mineral oil and pointing out the harm it can do by robbing the body of fat-soluble vitamins. To my knowledge, no one has studied the effect of rubbing mineral oil on an infant's skin; yet I feel that this practice should be condemned on circumstantial evidence.

If a baby oil is needed, any good salad oil such as peanut, corn, soybean, or olive, perhaps with a drop of perfume added, serves the purpose.

How much should babies be protected from bacteria? A report published recently told of the number of hemorrhages occurring in infants 6 to 10 days old. In a New York City hospital it was found that infants kept under the most sterile conditions possible suffered many times more hemorrhages than did a similar number of babies born at home. Vitamin K, produced by bacteria in the intestines, had prevented hemorrhages in the infants born at home, whereas the more protected babies had obtained so few bacteria that little or no vitamin K was supplied them.

A study which has always amused me was made some years ago of two groups of preschool children in New York City. One was a group of underprivileged children from the slums. The other group was of children from well-to-do homes. Records were kept over a period of years of all the diseases and infections suffered by the youngsters. It was found that the children from the slums had far fewer illnesses than did the privileged children.

The youngsters from the slums had been exposed to so many bacteria that they had built up sufficient antibodies to withstand further onslaughts of these bacteria. Antibodies are produced to fight bacteria only after the bacteria have gained access to the body. The children from the well-to-do homes had been so protected that their bodies had had little chance to build up defense mechanisms. Inoculations and vaccinations are nothing more than injections of dead or half-dead bacteria designed to stimulate the production of antibodies capable of destroying those specific bacteria later, if the child should be attacked by them.

I recently had lunch with a pediatrician who is the father of four beautiful little girls. He was laughing over his change of attitude toward bacteria. "With our first baby," he said, "we sterilized everything in sight and didn't allow anyone to come near her. With each child we sterilized less and less. Now we sterilize almost nothing and show our baby to everyone who will look at her, except, of course, someone with a virulent infection. We figure the sooner she builds up antibodies, the better."

The realization that bacteria, introduced a few at a time, can be valuable may help many young mothers to relax and enjoy their motherhood far more than women have in the past.

The pendulum swings. Because of the tremendous amount of research in all fields of infant care, the convictions of today are not necessarily those of tomorrow. Yet change, annoying though it may seem at times, is usually progress, and progress we all want.

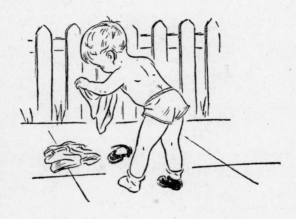

CHAPTER 15

YOUR BABY STARTS TO EAT

I CANNOT help feeling that the current practice of giving a 6- or 8-week-old infant practically every food except chili con carne, beer, and pretzels is definitely wrong. Since I almost skipped a generation before being able to have a family of my own, I have witnessed the entire swing of the pendulum in this respect. When I worked in the diet kitchen of the baby wards at Bellevue Hospital in New York City, we gave infants of 4 months and older 1 teaspoon or more of finely ground and steamed liver, an unheard-of thing prior to that time. At the baby clinics where I later worked, we suggested in the most tactful tone to mothers that they might start giving cooked cereal, mashed banana, and hard-cooked egg yolk to their 5-month-old infants. The mothers were often horrified: the babies were too young to be fed.

In contrast, I had lunch with a group of young mothers when Barbara, our little girl, was 6 months old. As we observed each other's babies, each probably thinking how much prettier her own was than the others, the mothers exclaimed repeatedly in amazement, "Barbara has never been given solid food!" They apparently assumed that a baby to be healthy must be fed solid foods early.

Years ago infants were not fed solids until they were 10 or 12 months old, and then only tiny bites from the family table. The practice of starting solids earlier and earlier came with advances in the study of nutrition. It was first realized that milk was deficient in iron; accordingly egg yolk, liver, and cereal were given to make up the deficiency. The next realization was that formulas and breast milk were both inadequate in the B vitamins; and cereal was introduced still earlier to supply them. Studies showed that infants who were fed solids early and thus obtained some of the nutrients lacking in the formula or breast milk thrived more than did infants given inadequate formulas of diluted milk and refined sugar. Advances in nutrition are now such, however, that every baby today should receive an adequate formula even during the first month, or before solid foods are given. Supplements can also make up for the deficiencies of breast milk; thus extremely early introduction of solids is no longer necessary.

Is the baby who is fed solids early benefited nutritionally? Since the argument for early feeding of solids is supposedly a nutritional one, let us analyze what an infant gains in nutrients by being put on three meals a day.

A neighbor of mine, a fine, conscientious mother, is gradually being indoctrinated with my ideas. Although she has an excellent pediatrician, she plies me with questions concerning infant feeding, has watched me mix formulas, and is not averse to imitating my procedures. Since her baby had had pneumonia and several colds, she first added 50 milligrams of vitamin C to each bottle of his formula. She next added blackstrap molasses and was quickly convinced of its value because his faulty elimination was corrected and his color improved. To put yeast in a baby's formula seemed drastic to her, but since my child thrived on it, she tried adding a small amount. Her baby started sleeping throughout the night for the first time and was less irritable during the day. She now thinks yeast is marvelous and should be given to all infants. She is quite proud, however, that her baby has been on three meals a day from the time he was barely 2 months old. Since she started to feed him, he has rarely taken as much as 24 ounces of formula daily; our baby, at the same age, consistently took 40 ounces.

When he was 5 months old, I asked her exactly what he ate during one particular day. On that day I watched her give him his midday meal. For breakfast he had 1 tablespoon of a canned baby cereal and ½ egg yolk. For lunch he ate, by generous estimate, about 1 tablespoon each of the following canned baby foods: beef and liver "soup" (undiluted), carrots, peas, and applesauce. His evening meal consisted of 2 tablespoons of canned vegetables with bacon and cereal and 1 tablespoon of canned peaches. Her selection of foods, I think you will agree, is as good as that given to most infants.

On pages 166 and 167 is the analysis of the food which her baby ate (the figures for the canned foods were obtained from the companies selling them) contrasted with the bottle of formula he would have taken if the foods had not been given him.

As you study these tables, you will see that if the baby had been given 8 ounces more of formula instead of the three meals, he would have received almost four times more protein, ten times more calcium, twice as much iron, three times as much vitamin B_1, four times as much vitamin B_2, twice as much niacin, and twenty times as much vitamin C. He obtained 2,401 more units of vitamin A from his meals, however, than he would have from his formula. This amount could have been obtained more easily and less expensively from 2 drops of vitamin-A concentrate. The advantage of the formula over solids becomes even more obvious when the nutrients gained in a 3-month period are considered.

The analysis does not show many nutrients which the formula would have supplied in far greater amounts than did the foods actually eaten. Few foods are so rich in trace minerals as are yeast, milk, and particularly blackstrap molasses. Yeast is also an excellent source of the B vitamins, pantothenic acid, para aminobenzoic acid, biotin, choline, inositol, vitamin B_6, and nucleic and adenylic acids, whereas blackstrap molasses supplies still more B vitamins, particularly pantothenic acid and inositol. Of the canned baby foods, only canned liver is rich in these particular nutrients.

This mother spent 35 minutes in feeding her baby lunch or over 1 hour a day in giving the three meals. She wrecked a good portion of an egg and opened seven cans of prepared baby foods, which represent a considerable financial outlay especially if one considers the amount spent in the course of 2 or 3 months. Certainly one could not say that the baby enjoyed the meal I

Formula He Did Not Take (8 ounces)	Measurement or weight	Protein grams	Calcium mg.	Iron mg.	Vitamin A units
Evaporated milk	4 ounces or 130 grams	9.1	315.9	.2	520
Vegetable cooking water	4 ounces	—	—	*	—
1 teaspoon yeast, rounded	10 grams	4.6	10	1.8	—
Blackstrap molasses	1 teaspoon	—	80	3.2	—
Vitamin C	50 milligrams	—	—	—	—
Total		13.7	405.9	5.2	520

Food Actually Eaten

BREAKFAST					
Cereal	1 tablespoon	.75	14	1.9	—
Egg yolk	½ yolk	1.6	14.7	.7	321
DINNER					
Beef and liver soup	1 tablespoon	.4	2.1	.2	391
Carrots	1 tablespoon	.08	3.3	.02	1,520
Peas	1 tablespoon	.4	1.9	.14	58
Applesauce	1 tablespoon	.02	.4	.04	3
SUPPER					
Vegetables with bacon and cereal	2 tablespoons	.26	2.4	.06	526
Peaches	1 tablespoon	.04	.7	.03	103
Total for entire day		3.55	39.5	3.09	2,922
Total intake in 40 ounces of formula and no food		68.5	2,029.5	26	2,600
Total intake with 3 meals and 24 ounces of formula		44.65	1,256.2	18.69	4,481
Nutrients gained in 1 day if no solids were fed		23.85	773.3	7.31	
Nutrients gained in 90 days if no solids were fed		2,146.5	69,597	657.9	

mg. = milligrams.
— Indicates that food contains none of the nutrient in question.
* Indicates that no figures are available but food may be a good source of the nutrient.

Formula He Did Not Take (8 ounces)	Measurement or weight	Vitamin B₁ mg.	Vitamin B₂ mg.	Niacin mg.	Vitamin C mg.
Evaporated milk	4 ounces or 130 grams	.07	.46	.3	—
Vegetable cooking water	4 ounces	*	*	*	*
1 teaspoon yeast, rounded	10 grams	.97	.54	3.6	—
Blackstrap molasses	1 teaspoon	.01	.02	*	—
Vitamin C	50 milligrams	—	—	—	50
Total		1.05	1.02	3.9	50

Food Actually Eaten

BREAKFAST

Cereal	1 tablespoon	.06	.05	1.2	—
Egg yolk	½ yolk	.03	.05	—	—

DINNER

Beef and liver soup	1 tablespoon	.002	.007	.17	.13
Carrots	1 tablespoon	.002	.005	.06	.09
Peas	1 tablespoon	.06	.045	.15	1.7
Applesauce	1 tablespoon	.001	.001	.006	.02

SUPPER

Vegetables with bacon and cereal	2 tablespoons	.22 †	.114 †	.10 †	.18
Peaches	1 tablespoon	.001	.002	.09	.27
Total for entire day		.376	.274	1.776	2.39

Total intake in 40 ounces of formula and no food		5.25	5.10	19.5	250
Total intake with 3 meals and 24 ounces of formula		3.526	3.334	13.476	152.39
Nutrients gained in 1 day if no solids were fed		1.724	1.766	6.024	97.61
Nutrients gained in 90 days if no solids were fed		155.16	158.94	542.16	874.3

† Brewers' yeast is added to this particular brand, which accounts for the increased amounts of vitamins B₁, B₂, and niacin.

watched him eat; there was the usual pushing the food out of the mouth and the mother's forcing it back again. When the meal was completed, the baby's face, bib, high chair, a portion of the floor and wall, and his dishes all had to be washed. Such expense and effort would be worth while, of course, if the baby enjoyed his meals and/or gained nutritionally from them.

Other supposed arguments for early feeding of solids. It is frequently argued that early feeding of solids is necessary in order to accustom the infant to the flavor and texture of many different foods; that a child who is fed solids early will less often develop feeding problems than one fed later.

In all probability, exactly the opposite of these arguments is true. An infant's taste buds are only slightly developed during his first 6 months; unless a flavor is unusually pungent, he probably fails to differentiate one taste from another. If he learns to enjoy a flavor, he probably does so when he is 6 or 8 months old even though that particular food was given him at 6 weeks. Anyone who argues that stuffing a 3-month-old baby with spinach guarantees that he will enjoy it when he is 3 years old has, in my opinion, been around too few children to know them.

Early feeding of solids often delays a child's getting acquainted with a variety of textures. One frequently finds children 2 and 3 years old who will eat nothing except canned baby foods. Solids were given them so early that only foods of smooth textures could be allowed; they became so accustomed to puréed foods that later they refused foods with coarser textures.

Experiments have shown that the giving of solids too early can cause feeding problems. Dr. Rowan-Legg (ref. 2, p. 142) points out that infants fed when too young frequently develop an antagonism to spoons which may persist for months. Similarly infants offered cups too early, especially if the bottle is taken away from them against their will, may dislike the cup to such an extent that they will refuse to drink milk. Serious health problems as well as feeding problems can thus arise.

If for any reason solid foods must be given early, dilute them with milk or formula or fruit juice, and allow the baby to take them from a bottle (p. 146).

Late feeding is easier. Introducing solid foods when a baby is 6 or 8 months old is easier for both the mother and child. During a baby's first few months he instinctively forces objects from his mouth. By the time most babies are 6 months old, their mouthing instincts are well developed, and from then on almost every object small enough to go into the mouth is put into it. This eagerness for new mouthing experience makes the introduction of solid foods a joy. Furthermore, most healthy infants from 6 to 18 months old have appetites like little pigs, and everything offered them is usually eagerly devoured.

When to introduce solid foods. Since no two babies are alike, the time to introduce solid foods varies with each child. One baby may be ready for solids months before another. Dr. Rowan-Legg (ref. 2, p. 142) stresses that foods should never be introduced by age but only when the baby is still hungry *after* the formula is given. Such a time may be when he is 3 months old or not until he is 6 or 8 months old. This pediatrician also states that under no circumstances should a certain amount of food be specified, such as 2 tablespoons of cereal or vegetable; and that feeding should be stopped immediately when the infant shows he does not want more.

It seems to me there are seven rules which may guide you as to when and how solids should be introduced. Let us list them separately:

1. Give solid foods only after your baby has been nursed or has taken his formula.

2. Do not try to feed him from a spoon until he is strong enough to sit comfortably and hold himself erect in a high chair for the duration of the meal.

3. Offer food from time to time, and watch your baby's reaction. Start regular meals only when he has sufficient control of his tongue and throat to shift the food easily to the back of the mouth and to swallow it without difficulty. If he forces food

from his mouth, he is not ready to be fed. Forcing food out of the mouth, however, is different from merely spilling it.

4. Your baby should be eager to take the food from the spoon when it is not touching his lips. If he opens his mouth in birdlike fashion and leans forward to get the food, he is probably ready to be fed.

5. The child should be old enough to be allowed foods of varying textures, such as soft curds of cottage cheese or uncooked wheat germ moistened with milk.

6. Even in case your baby enjoys the food enough to eat it in quantity, do not allow him more than 1 or 2 teaspoons the first time the food is introduced. Wait and see how he tolerates it. A small amount cannot upset him severely.

7. The baby should express interest throughout the meal. Feeding should be stopped at the first sign of displeasure.

When the formula is adequate or the breast milk is of high quality, and when supplements are given to make up the deficiencies of either, the point to remember is this: *the purpose of introducing solid food is not a nutritional one*. Unless great caution is used, the infant's diet may become worse rather than better when solids are given him. The purpose of introducing solids is to allow your baby to learn to eat just as you allow him to learn to walk; he is preparing for the future.

How to introduce solid foods. The important question is how to introduce foods rather than which foods to give first or when to introduce them. Obtain several demitasse spoons, avoiding large baby spoons until the child is perhaps 1 year old. One demitasse spoon is a must; it is convenient to have three or four. Let the baby play with a spoon; tie it to his high chair or cradle gym; let him finger it, mouth it, and use it for teething. Only after the spoon has become an old friend should it be used for feeding him.

One reason solids are often forced on infants is that the foods given are usually canned baby foods. You have gone to the effort of buying and heating them and wrapping a bib or diaper around the baby's neck, only to find that meal after meal he may little

more than taste them. Perhaps you are swamped with work, and
the budget is stretched to the limit; naturally you resent the
time and money you have spent. After you have offered your
baby such foods as cereal or liver soup or puréed spinach a few
times and he has refused them, there is nothing to do but throw
them out since neither you nor your husband can stand them.
Under such circumstances, especially if you happen to be tired
enough to feel irritable, it is quite understandable that you may
decide that the baby jolly well has to eat or else. You are off to
the races, but on the wrong track.

It seems to me that our grandmothers had the right idea about
feeding the babies from the family table. At least their technic
has worked out well with our children. Since our little girl was
about 3 months old, she has enjoyed sitting in her high chair
near our dining-room table while we eat. As soon as she was old
enough to pick up objects, a demitasse spoon was tied to one side
of her high chair and a small plastic cup to the other. These
"toys" she played with, mouthed, and chewed on.

When she was about 4 months old, I began offering her nibbles
of any of our food which was soft in texture or could be mashed
easily into sufficiently small particles not to choke her. At first,
she rarely took the food; she sometimes accepted it and then
forced it out of her mouth with an expression which looked as if
she had been given rat poison. During her fifth month, however,
she began taking almost every food offered her. By the time she
was 7 months old, she had tasted the following foods: a variety of
cooked cereals; uncooked wheat germ with milk; several cream
soups; brown and converted rice and whole buckwheat; every
kind of cooked squash; mashed, baked, creamed, and au gratin
potatoes; baked sweet potatoes and yams; cooked tomatoes,
steamed carrots, parsnips, kohlrabi, tiny new turnips, and broc-
coli; applesauce, scraped raw apple, very ripe mashed raw
peaches, apricots, bananas, avocados, and tomatoes; watermelon,
cantaloupe, honeydew and Persian melons; hard-cooked egg yolk,
macaroni and cheese, cottage cheese, bits of American and Swiss
cheese, and crisp bacon; tiny cubes of kidney and sautéed liver,

bites of ground round steak and slivers of fish and chicken; the sauces from a number of such dishes as beef hash, Spanish rice and spaghetti with tomatoes; custard, yogurt, junket, and peanut butter; and sips of yeast mixed with pineapple or grapefruit juice. She chewed on raw carrot, turnip and kohlrabi sticks to help in teething.

By using this method, a mother needs to spend no extra money and almost no time in preparing foods for the baby. Therefore there is no temptation to force foods which are not wanted. The baby becomes acquainted with a wide variety of foods and textures at a time when he has eager interest in both. When this procedure is followed, most babies will show that they are ready for three meals some time between the ages of 6 and 9 months.

Learning to drink from a cup. In my opinion, the main purpose in teaching a baby to drink from a cup early is first to prevent his mother from neglecting his orange juice, which is difficult to strain so that it will pass readily through small nipple holes, and, second, to accustom him to the flavor of yeast in juice.

Before you offer your baby any liquid from a lovely sterling cup, drink out of it yourself. In most cases, such cups impart a metallic flavor which your baby will probably not enjoy any more than you would. A clear plastic cup or tiny pitcher is usually much more satisfactory. A trick which works well at first is to hold a sauce dish under the baby's chin and the cup as he drinks; then pour the spilled juice back into the cup.

I see no reason why a mother should be proud that her baby can drink milk from a cup when 5 or 6 months old; she could as well expect him to conjugate verbs at this age. Milk should be taken from a bottle as long as the baby will take it.

Procedures which are easiest for the baby and which do not antagonize him are also the easiest for you, his mother.

CHAPTER 16

YOUR BABY GOES ON THREE MEALS

MOST mothers work far too hard at feeding their babies during the first 2 years; they go to too much trouble, spend too much time and money on food, and worry over it too much. During the next 2 years—and multiples of the next 2—many of them do exactly the opposite. Perhaps if baby feeding could be accepted in a somewhat relaxed manner, enough energy would be left over for more careful vigilance later. Your baby can be well nourished without your slaving over his meals or even worrying about them.

When you use the tastes-from-the-family-table method to introduce foods, no work is involved. Eventually, however, your baby will want sufficient quantities of food to constitute meals. Take it easy and start by giving him one meal a day. If he gets hungry during the night, give him his first meal in the evening. In case he sleeps soundly, begin with any meal which is most convenient for you. In a week or so, start giving him a second meal, and a few days later, a third.

What foods shall we give the baby? The menus for your baby's meals can be quite conventional ones. His breakfast should depend on what you are serving the other members of your family. If you squeeze oranges for them, give the baby his juice at breakfast; otherwise give him fruit, such as applesauce or mashed banana. Use only unrefined cereals for your family and cook them in milk so that they will be suitable to give your baby. Wheat germ with middlings is probably the best cooked cereal available, but any whole-grain cereal is satisfactory, especially if you add wheat germ to it. Since bran becomes extremely soft when soaked a few minutes, the cereal need not be ground especially fine. Avoid using the baby cereals which have synthetic vitamins B$_1$, B$_2$, and niacin added to them. Your baby needs all the B vitamins, not just a few of them.

If you are not serving cooked cereal to the family, you might give the baby uncooked wheat germ mixed with milk or stirred into his fruit. Remember, however, that wheat germ is quite laxative; use it cautiously until you know how your baby tolerates it.

In case you are boiling or poaching eggs for the family, cook one until the yolk is firm and give the baby the yolk instead of cereal or in addition to it. Scrambled eggs and omelet are probably suitable for a healthy baby 6 or 8 months old provided they are cooked thoroughly. Uncooked egg white can cause an allergy or a biotin deficiency (p. 204), but it contains good protein and vitamin B$_2$, and it need not be avoided if properly cooked.

Most babies enjoy crisp bacon, but care must be taken to break it into tiny pieces to avoid danger of choking. Toast should be crisp for the same reason; it should be made only of 100 per cent whole-wheat or whole-rye bread or of wheat-germ bread. By the time the baby is 1 year old, he can be given bite-size pieces of waffles, hot cakes, and French toast provided they are made with ingredients which can build health and are served only with butter (or margarine) and perhaps a fruit sauce. Few foods can have so much brewers' yeast, blackstrap, wheat germ, and powdered milk added and still be delicious as can waffles and hot cakes.

The baby's lunch and dinner should supply some food containing protein: egg yolk if none was given for breakfast; cottage cheese, mashed cream cheese, or shredded and moistened American or Swiss cheese; a cream soup, preferably fortified with powdered milk; a meat such as liver, kidney, heart, or brains; or a dessert made with powdered milk such as junket, custard, or thick yogurt (p. 175). In fact, it is sound nutrition to give a baby two protein-containing foods at a meal, such as cottage cheese and yogurt or custard at noon, and a cream soup and meat at night. No more than one vegetable need be served at either meal.

If you do not give him a high-protein dessert, let him have fruit or skip dessert entirely.

Whenever you need to heat chilled foods for a baby, instead of using a cooking utensil, put the foods into small heat-resistant custard cups and set them in a pan of warm water.

Stress the foods which supply the nutrients he may be lacking. The foods you may need to stress will depend upon what sources of nutrients, if any, you are adding to his milk, what supplements you give him, and the amount of milk he is taking. If yeast, blackstrap molasses, and vegetable water are used in the formula, and if wheat-germ oil is given as a supplement, the baby is already getting many times more iron, B vitamins, and vitamin E than he can get from any amount of cereal he could eat; therefore cereals need not be particularly stressed unless you take his bottle away from him. As soon as he begins to drink from a cup, he may refuse milk with yeast in it because of the odor which was not noticeable in the formula. In this case, or if wheat-germ oil is discontinued, cereals may be his only source of vitamin E and the B vitamins and should be given daily or twice daily in as large quantities as he will eat.

If you have given the baby an evaporated-milk formula, your pediatrician may recommend that you now change to certified or homogenized milk. You should, however, continue to add the yeast, blackstrap, and vitamin C. Vegetables must now be relied upon to supply the minerals formerly obtained from vegetable water; hence vegetables become somewhat more important than before.

Since breast milk appears to support the growth of valuable intestinal bacteria more than cows' milk, it is undoubtedly wise to introduce yogurt (p. 30) early into the diet of the bottle-fed baby and to give it frequently, even daily if desired. A thick yogurt can be prepared by beating 1½ cups of powdered skim milk with 2 cups of water and 3 tablespoons of previously prepared yogurt or yogurt culture; * to this mixture 1 quart of water

* Can be obtained from many companies marketing yogurt or from the Trappist Monks, La Trappe, Quebec, Canada.

and a large can of evaporated milk are added; it can be poured into glasses set in warm water, incubated at approximately 110 degrees F. for 3 hours, or until thick, and then chilled. Yogurt thus prepared can be kept for 1 week or more. It supplies not only valuable bacteria but twice as much protein as does ordinary milk or most commercial yogurt.

Do not let solid foods crowd out milk. When babies are put on three meals, their milk intake usually decreases markedly, sometimes to as little as 8 ounces a day. The mothers seem to be proud of the large amounts of canned foods the babies consume, yet they worry too little about the decreased milk intake.

Every baby under 1 year old, in my opinion, should receive each day a minimum of three bottles of milk, or 24 ounces, and preferably four bottles, or 32 ounces. Almost any infant not stuffed to the gills with canned baby foods will take this quantity. If 1 rounded teaspoon of yeast is added to each 8-ounce bottle of milk, four bottles would supply 54.8 grams of protein. When a baby's appetite is so satisfied with solids that his milk consumption drops to 8 ounces daily, he will receive 41 grams of protein less from his formula. To supply this deficit, he would have to eat daily more than 9 entire cans of beef and liver soup, 16 cans of beef broth with beef and barley, or 19 cans of lamb and vegetables with milk and cereal. To supply the deficit of calcium (975 milligrams) he would need to eat daily at least 45 cans of any one of these foods. Equally ridiculous figures can be arrived at if other baby foods are selected for comparison.

A criticism of canned baby foods. I believe that canned baby foods are given too early, too long, and too generously; it seems to me their nutritional value is tremendously overestimated. I do not, however, completely disapprove of them; their convenience is unquestioned. Most of the companies marketing canned baby foods make every effort to grow the foods on good soils, keep them free from poison sprays, and can them when fresh, using methods which will best preserve nutritive value. Canned and puréed vegetables are undoubtedly superior to vegetables which have been grown on poor soil, covered with poison sprays, shipped 3,000 miles, held for an unknown period in a market where they may be sprinkled or soaked in water, then taken home, perhaps peeled, soaked again, and boiled before being given to a baby. On the other hand, canned vegetables are not superior to those grown in soil rich in humus, freshly picked from your own garden, and prepared by methods known to preserve nutritive value.

If you read the labels on canned baby foods, you may be impressed by the number of foods to which wheat germ and yeast are added. The quantity of vitamins obtained from such amounts of yeast or wheat germ, however, is small indeed. The labels also show that many of these foods contain cornstarch, farina, polished rice, "wheat" flour (meaning white), and arrowroot. Your baby's appetite should not be satisfied with these devitalized ingredients.

The advantages of preparing your baby's food yourself. I remarked to my pediatrician that I would not enjoy eating canned foods almost entirely and that I had no intention of putting my baby on a diet of them. He replied, "If I had my way, every mother would have a blender so that she could prepare foods for her baby from those cooked for the family." Many mothers besides myself have found his suggestion to be an excellent one.

In case blenders are new to you, they look like gadgets for making milk shakes but have revolving knives which reduce solids to a paste or liquid. They are sold under various names such as blenders, liquefiers, osterizers, and Fletcherizers. Such a machine is well worth buying if you can possibly afford it. In selecting a blender, however, choose one with a base which can be unscrewed; at times you may wish to blend only a small amount of food, which is more easily removed from the bottom than the top.

The advantages of using blended foods rather than canned ones are numerous. You get better food for far less money. Quickly cooked and blended fresh vegetables certainly surpass in flavor and color any canned food you can buy. If you prepare your vegetables carefully, their nutritive value is undoubtedly greater than that of canned foods which, necessarily heated to high temperatures, lose considerable carotene, folic acid, and vitamins B_1 and C. Furthermore, canned foods are stored for unknown lengths of time, causing further losses. Even when fresh foods are quickly cooked, blended, frozen, stored a short time, and then reheated, the nutritive losses are probably less than in canned foods.

Another advantage of using a blender is that you can prepare for your baby any number of foods which are not available in cans; for example, cooked meats such as heart, kidney, brains, and chicken livers; or uncooked apples, pears, berries, guavas, carrots, and sweet bell peppers. If the baby does not drink orange juice well from a cup, an orange and some of the white part of the rind (for vitamin P) can be blended and served the baby as a sauce. In fact, you can prepare for the baby almost any raw fruit or vegetable or even certain raw meats, which some pediatricians recommend highly.

Few foods, for instance, have higher nutritive value than have brains, yet so many mothers are squeamish about preparing them that most babies never taste them. If the brains are washed quickly and frozen in an ice tray, then sliced and blended with milk or tomato juice, the texture and appearance are so changed that few mothers object to them. The brains may be cooked for the baby but are superior nutritionally when given raw.

Using the blender, I prepare a liver paste which our family thinks is so delicious that it is usually eaten before the baby gets more than a taste. I steam an onion and three or four carrots until almost tender, then add 1 pound of calves' liver, and steam the food about 7 minutes longer. (Lamb liver can be used.) After the food is blended, I salt it to taste and store it in small jars in the refrigerator or freezer. Whenever I make such dishes as kidney creole or stew using heart meat, I blend enough of them to have several meals for the baby. Every mother who owns a blender has her own pet recipes which she can convert into baby foods.

If you have your own garden, the variety of foods which can be blended is almost endless. In addition to vegetables customarily given to babies, you can blend quickly cooked chard, kale, beet tops, tampala, tiny new turnip tops, small turnips, parsnips, kohlrabi, every variety of squash, both red and green cabbage, and bell peppers. You can also blend almost any raw vegetable which has a pleasant flavor, such as fresh peas, kohlrabi, carrots, ripe bell pepper or pimiento, or tiny beets or turnips, or various combinations of several vegetables.

So little liquid need be used that most blended foods can be somewhat thicker than canned baby foods. When a food is too juicy, wheat germ, powdered milk, or pablum can be added to thicken it. Since many greens such as spinach and kale contain oxalic acid which can combine with calcium and prevent it from reaching the blood, it is wise to add 1 teaspoon or more of powdered milk for each serving whenever you prepare leafy vegetables for the baby. If the baby has given up his bottle and is not getting enough yeast or milk, both yeast and powdered skim milk can be blended with any number of foods.

The easiest method of preparing food for the baby is to cook nourishing food for the family and to blend some of it for the baby. Your vegetables should be fresh, washed quickly but thoroughly, and steamed only until tender in the least amount of water possible. If a vegetable is dry, such as carrots cooked without water, 2 or 3 tablespoons of milk can be put into the blender first. When a little water is left from steaming the vegetable, it can be used instead. Naturally moist foods, such as greens, need no added liquid. Since blending the food takes only a minute, it can be served immediately. If more convenient, however, blend the food, and store it in the refrigerator or freeze it. For example, foods left from your own meals may be blended separately, or several vegetables may be blended with meat, then chilled or frozen. When only bits of several foods are left, they may be blended and put into separate compartments of an ice tray; a cube of frozen food is usually about the amount needed for a baby.

Another advantage of using a blender is that you know exactly what goes into the food, and such ingredients as cornstarch and white flour used in canned baby foods may be omitted. Furthermore, as your baby grows older, he should become accustomed to coarser textures; foods can then be blended less thoroughly.

Before you have actually prepared your own baby foods, it may seem to be too much trouble. The food can be blended quickly, however, and the blender need only to be rinsed. A mother of an 18-month-old child said to me recently, "I bought a lot of canned baby foods, but I like the blended foods so well that I have never opened one can." Many mothers find themselves doing the same thing.

Shall we give the baby crackers and toast? The accepted practice of giving a 6- to 18-month-old child crackers and melba toast between meals is of questionable value. The argument that these foods, if hard and dry, help to develop the jaws probably has no scientific basis. Although exercising your arms may cause you to develop bulging muscles, it probably does not increase the size of your arm bone one iota. A well-developed mouth is one in which the bone structure is normal, not one where the jaw muscles are massive. When animals are undersupplied with vitamin C, their teeth loosen; if they are then given hard food to chew, the harder the food and the more of it given, the more crooked their teeth become.

If the mother has the conviction that crackers and toast are valuable, and if she allows her child to chew them as much as he likes, his appetite for more nourishing foods can easily be destroyed. I recently observed a boy of 18 months, pale, whiny, irritable, with poor posture and poorer appetite, who, almost every waking minute, was chewing white toast, stuffed into his hands by the mother who could not stand his fretful whining. At mealtimes, the child ate little except what was forced into his mouth; his appetite had already been ruined.

Giving a child crackers is but a short step from the cookie habit. Many 2- to 4-year-old children would almost live on crackers and cookies if allowed to do so. In case the mother happens to be tired and perhaps busy with a new baby, the plea for "quacker, quacker, mo quacker," especially if demanded in a shrill, irritable, or whiny voice, can wear her down to the extent that she temporarily cares little whether the child's appetite is ruined or even his teeth fall out provided he will only shut up and leave her alone. When a child has never been given crackers except at meals or definite midmeals, this problem rarely arises.

Letting your baby chew toast or crackers between meals is undeniably a messy habit. The amount of nutrients he actually gains, if any, is too small to be of value. Most of the melba toast and crackers available are made of white flour, refined sugar usually being added to enhance the flavor. Even most crackers made with some whole-wheat flour, such as graham crackers, also contain white flour and refined sugar.

When a baby is teething, sticks of celery, carrots, kohlrabi, and raw foods of similar texture are excellent for him to chew. Plastic teething bags, filled with distilled water which can be chilled, also appear to be helpful. The child's jaw muscles, however, will develop without any help from the manufacturers of crackers and melba toast.

When shall junior foods be started? A pediatrician told me his answer to this question was, "When your child is ready for junior foods, he is ready for senior foods. Let him eat from the family table." The age at which a child will accept pieces of food rather than puréed foods varies with the development of the child and the textures of food already given him. Many foods with coarse textures, such as the curds of cottage cheese, tiny pieces of Swiss or American cheese, and meat cut perhaps into ⅛-inch cubes, should be given early, between the fifth and eighth month. When the introduction of various textures is delayed, a child sometimes rebels against the food, and both feeding problems and health problems arise.

Make your schedule suit your own needs. You may say, remembering that the bottle should always come before a meal: "This all sounds fine, but it just doesn't work out. I can give the baby his bottle before breakfast; that's easy. But I give him his breakfast 2 hours later; he takes his morning nap soon afterward and wants his bottle before he goes to sleep; that bottle must come after he eats rather than before. For lunch I have a salad and sandwich; he can't eat that, and it can't be blended very well. Sometimes I could feed him from the family table at dinner, but if I stop to feed him, I can't enjoy my own meal. Besides the baby spills too much food on the new dining-room rug, or my husband gets home so late that I want the baby in bed before dinner is served."

There is nothing ironclad about the suggestions that I have made. Arrange your schedule to suit yourself. In fact, schedules have been purposely omitted throughout the book. Any schedule should be worked out co-operatively by yourself and your baby.

If your child takes a nap immediately after your meal, perhaps you can serve his meal earlier or make it a small one. When your lunch consists of foods he cannot eat, give him cottage cheese, mashed banana, or wheat germ with milk. In case he eats a hearty evening meal, he should be fed early so that he will want his bottle before going to sleep; to eat with the family at that meal may be undesirable. In any case, the parents need consideration as well as the baby.

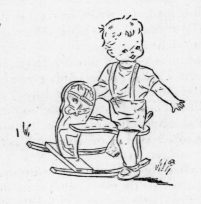

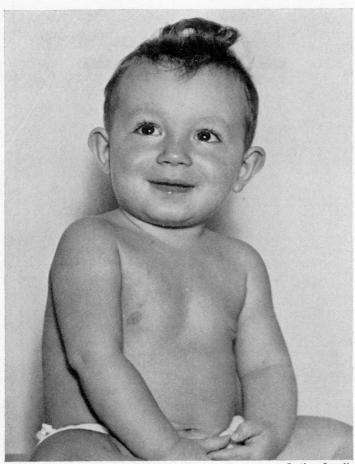

Regardless of family resemblances, a child's eyes should be widely spaced and there should be width of bone from the outer part of the eyes to the ears. The chest, the forehead and the middle and lower thirds of the face should likewise be wide. Good muscular development should be evident by the flatness of the abdomen which forms a straight line with the chest.

CHAPTER 17

MILK IS STILL YOUR CHILD'S
MOST IMPORTANT FOOD

IN MY opinion taking the bottle away from the baby too soon leads to more problems between the ages of 1 to 3 or 4 years than do all other causes put together. If a baby enjoys his bottle, and if yeast, blackstrap molasses, and vitamin C are added to the milk, and if supplements are given to supply vitamins A, D, and E, his diet is fairly complete without anything else. Even if such a child's other eating habits are faulty indeed, he will probably still be a healthy, beautiful child.

When eating problems arise, a mother's knowledge that her child is getting his essential nutrients from his bottle and supplements is so comforting and reassuring that its value to her cannot be overestimated. Furthermore, in case your child becomes ill, he is often willing to drink from a bottle though he may refuse all other food; if he is not allowed a bottle, he may eat little or nothing for the duration of his illness.

When the bottle is taken away, the amount of milk the child drinks almost invariably decreases. Frequently a child will refuse to drink a mixture of milk, yeast, and molasses from a cup. His diet often becomes deficient in protein, the B vitamins, calcium, iron, and many trace minerals. When the bottle is taken away, therefore, dozens of problems can arise with sickening speed.

Advantages of giving milk from a bottle. The advantages of continuing the bottle can best be pointed out by specific examples. About a year ago I spent a day with a fine conscientious mother and her beautiful 10-month-old boy, a happy, smiling youngster, the picture of health. His bone structure was excellent; his chest was broad and round; his abdomen was held in with firm muscles; and his little back was so straight that he held himself like a king.

I did not see the child again until 8 months later. Although the mother warned me on the phone that she and her husband were worried about him, I could scarcely believe my eyes when she removed his clothing and placed him before me. Except for the lower ribs, his chest bones were flat and caved in. His stomach protruded badly, although it appeared abnormally large in contrast to the sunken, misshapen chest. Even though he was not thin, his little shoulders were rounded, and the shoulder blades stood out in "angel wings." The soles of his feet were as flat as sheets of paper, and on the inside of each foot a bone protruded at the place where there should have been an arch. I felt sick. How could I have let this happen to the child of a personal friend?

The boy appeared to be deficient in protein and vitamin D. The mother assured me he was getting egg and cereal at breakfast, a can of meat at noon, and cottage cheese at his evening meal; that she rarely forgot to give him his cod-liver-oil concentrate; and that she gave it in adequate amounts. What then could account for the faulty chest formation and for muscles so flabby that they could not hold the shoulder blades, the stomach, and the arches of the feet in place? I was completely baffled until the mother chanced to ask, "Do you suppose it's because he won't drink milk?"

When the baby was 9 months old, her pediatrician had told her it was time for him to take milk from a cup. The child had not objected seriously except that he refused all milk for 2 weeks; the doctor had warned her that was to be expected. Since then he had taken only 2 or 3 ounces of milk at each meal even though she had done her best to have him take more. Now and then when her husband did not eat breakfast at home, however, she gave the baby a morning bottle so that she could sleep later. He took it eagerly, showing that he still enjoyed drinking milk in that manner. Will this child's chest, shoulders, abdomen, and feet become normal again? I do not know, but it is certain that his abnormalities could have been easily, so easily, prevented.

Few children can eat enough eggs, meats, and cheese to fulfill their protein requirements adequately; they must also have the protein from milk. Remember that a quart of milk supplies 33 grams of protein; to obtain that same amount of protein, a child would have to eat 6½ eggs or about ½ pound of meat or cottage cheese. Furthermore, no amount of vitamin D can substitute for the bone-building calcium which only milk supplies in the quantity needed.

Instead of this case history I could have selected one of hundreds much like it or another where the cause was the same but the resulting deviations from health differed. Since muscles are made of protein, they lose their turgor, or strength, whenever protein is inadequate; the number of little potbellies, rounded shoulders, and flat feet which can be seen in any nursery school is appalling, even though the children come from well-to-do homes. Bones cannot develop normally without adequate calcium; faulty bone structure seems to be almost the rule rather than the exception.

When the bottle is taken away, a child may suffer from a series of infections because his body cannot produce sufficient numbers of antibodies and white blood cells when his protein intake is inadequate. Middle-ear infections, sinusitis, bronchitis, pneumonia, skin infections, or perhaps even a kidney infection may occur. Sometimes allergies appear which might have been prevented if the protein had been more generously supplied. Frequently eczema results from the lack of any one of several B vitamins which would have been furnished by yeast if the bottle had been continued. Perhaps the problem is one of dehydration because too few liquids are taken without the bottle. Constipation or anemia may occur, resulting from the decreased supply of B vitamins or iron. Almost invariably when the intake of calcium and the B vitamins decreases, a child who may have had a sunny disposition becomes tense and irritable and sleeps less than he should. Such a child is both difficult to handle and difficult to live with and can wear down any mother's nerves.

If mothers could only foresee that these problems arise with unbelievable speed and depressing frequency, they would be less proud when their 6- or 7-month-old babies drink only from a cup. When the bottle is continued, such problems can be largely or entirely avoided.

A little girl almost 5 years old often comes to play with our son. She has been thin, pale, and irritable, a constant worry to her parents. A few days ago I noticed that she had suddenly put on weight, had color in her cheeks, and her disposition had improved almost unbelievably. I asked the mother what had brought about the change.

She answered in a whisper: "I wouldn't tell anyone except you, but for the last month I've been giving her three bottles a day, one when she wakes up in the morning, one before her nap, and one before bed. It's the only way I can get enough milk down her, and she won't take yeast or blackstrap unless it's mixed with milk and taken from the bottle."

An unusual case, yes. Aside from the child's health, however, the parents now have peace of mind for the first time in 2 or 3 years.

Between the extremes of 9 months and 5 years, there comes a time when the child will want to give up his bottle, and it is desirable for him to do so. That time varies with each child and should depend upon his general food habits, his health, his willingness to take yeast out of a glass, the quantity of milk he will drink from a cup and, of course, his own preference. In actual practice it usually depends not upon these important factors but upon the mother's attitude and the advice given her by her pediatrician.

Why are bottles given up? There are probably dozens of contributing factors which cause the babies themselves to give up their bottles. Usually, however, there is one chief reason: the child is stuffed so full of canned baby foods that there is no room for milk from bottle or cup. If the bottle is consistently given before solids are offered, and if the amounts of other food are held within reasonable limits, this problem does not arise.

On the other hand, why do mothers take bottles away from

their babies? The reason I took a bottle away from our son was that when he was 22 months old, he repeatedly removed the nipples. By the tenth or twelfth time I found the bed soaked with milk, I decided I'd had enough. If I had foreseen the problem, I could have used screw-top bottles with nipples which cannot be removed easily.

Many mothers take away the bottles because they get tired of washing and filling them. The problems which arise when the child's milk intake decreases usually cause the mother to spend many times more energy than she had hoped to save. Some mothers may wish to "economize" by not buying more bottles to replace those which athletic babies throw out of the crib and break. Such economy often proves false because abnormalities resulting from the less adequate diet may mean large medical and dental bills. When a baby breaks bottles by trying to play baseball with them, put him on a blanket or soft rug on the floor while he takes his milk.

How much milk does your child drink? If the highest degree of health is to be built with minimum effort, a child should drink 1 quart of milk daily. Almost any child or adult who is not drinking this amount of milk will at times suffer from deficiencies of calcium, protein, and vitamin B_2. A mistake many mothers make is in not knowing how much milk a child actually drinks.

Time and again mothers have assured me that their children drink "lots of milk—no problem there at all—they love milk." Yet these children frequently show symptoms which would not exist if the milk intake had been adequate. In such cases, I ask the mothers to mark a bottle of milk for each child and to observe during 1 week exactly how much he drinks daily. Usually when the mother reports to me, she is somewhat disturbed because she had found that the child is not drinking nearly as much milk as she thought he was.

A system of bottle marking which I have found convenient is to drop a small jar lid over the bottle after replacing the cap. I use lids from instant coffee jars. One company thoughtfully furnishes blue lids, another pink; hence even the sexes can be differentiated. Regardless of your method of marking the bottle, check your child's milk intake at least once each week and preferably daily.

Increasing the milk intake. Whenever your child fails day after day to drink 1 quart of milk, steps should be taken to rectify the situation. Urging him to drink more will do little or no good. Your method should be unknown to the child.

There are a number of tricks which can be used to increase the milk intake. Some children will drink more milk merely by being allowed to take it through a straw; others by being allowed to pour each glassful from a small pitcher; still others by using a variety of brightly colored cups and glasses. These devices are usually temporary but can be tried from time to time.

The best method, however, although a nuisance, is to mix powdered skim milk into each quart of fresh milk. Although many children enjoy the flavor of such fortified milk, some dislike it at first; hence it is usually wise to start by adding ¼ cup of powdered milk to 1 quart of fresh milk and to increase the amount gradually. The mixing can most easily be done with a blender, or liquefier. If 1 cup of fresh milk is poured into the blender, the motor started, and the powdered milk carefully dropped into the vortex created by the whirling liquid, no powder will stick to the edges, and the blender need only to be rinsed. This mixture is then stirred into the original quart of fresh milk.

Not long ago a mother told me she was extremely worried because her 20-month-old boy would not drink more than a glass of milk daily. Now she tells me that since she added ½ cup of powdered milk to his fresh milk, he has increased his daily intake to four glasses of 8 ounces each (2 quarts of milk). Another mother happily reported that her children had disliked their milk when she first added powdered milk to it. The preceding day, however, the family had eaten in a restaurant, and the children had not finished their milk. "It doesn't taste good like ours at home," they had said.

To incorporate more milk in your cooking is an obvious remedy; usually the child obtains too little milk by this method unless it is concentrated as is powdered or evaporated milk. If a child is still eating canned or blended foods, 1 teaspoon or more of powdered milk can be mixed with a serving of almost any cereal, vegetable, fruit, or meat. Canned or homemade cream soups are excellent if ½ cup or more of powdered milk is beaten into each pint of fresh milk used. Some children love the taste of yogurt. A thick yogurt (p. 175) can be prepared for them. Although it is undoubtedly best to avoid desserts except fruits, a milk dessert is justified in case the milk intake drops below normal.

The two desserts which can incorporate the most milk with the least amount of sugar are custards and junkets; blackstrap molasses, honey, or blended dates can be used instead of part or all of the sugar. Although children usually love these desserts, mothers often believe they are difficult to prepare. A junket can be made in about 3 minutes. Cooking a boiled custard is essentially the same as scrambling eggs and takes the same amount of time; the only difference is that you add sweetening, vanilla, and more milk. A ½-cup serving of either of these desserts, if made with powdered milk, can be equivalent to 12 ounces of fresh milk. Such junket is not watery but has the texture of a thick pudding. Prepared puddings and junket powders contain so much sugar that they cannot be recommended. If prepared junket is used, powdered milk should be beaten with half the milk in the recipe while the other half is being heated; ½ to 1 cup of powdered milk can also be stirred with the dry ingredients of any pudding.

Few cooking habits can increase the health of your entire family so much as the use of powdered milk. It can be added to cream sauces, gravies, meat loaves and patties, every milk drink, breads, waffles, hot cakes, cookies, and dozens of other foods. It is one of the least expensive foods which can be purchased, yet it supplies more nutrients than almost any other food. Recipes for foods fortified with powdered milk are given in *Let's Cook It Right* by Adelle Davis (New York: Harcourt, Brace and Company, 1947).

Almost an endless variety of milk drinks can be prepared. Older children can make such drinks themselves though perhaps they may mess up the kitchen a bit. Often they work out wonderful recipes. Powdered milk (¼ cup) can be beaten into 8 ounces of fresh orange juice (add a drop of vanilla) or pineapple, apricot, Concord grape, raspberry, or almost any other sweet juice. If you have a blender, delicious milk shakes and malted milks can be prepared by combining fresh, powdered and frozen milk with sweetened fruits, honey, molasses, maple syrup, or seeded dates. One mother I know, who has four beautiful children, serves them every afternoon milk shakes which are nothing more than tigers' milk (p. 3); she keeps a tray of milk frozen in her refrigerator at all times and blends the fresh, powdered, and frozen milk with yeast and blackstrap. She tells me her children love it. One of our favorites is fresh, powdered, and frozen milk blended with seeded dates. The resulting drink looks so much like a chocolate milk shake that you almost imagine it tastes like one. Cocoa and chocolate have been found to interfere with the utilization of protein and calcium in experimental animals and are probably not to be recommended for children.

Another trick, which I am not beyond using, is to increase the thirst for milk by serving salty foods: hot dogs, ham, liver sausage, salty cheeses, or potato chips. You may add a liberal amount of salt to your child's favorite food as you prepare it. Salty foods not only increase the milk intake but are excellent substitutes for candy and cookies. Regardless of how much you try to prevent it, sooner or later some thoughtless person will give your youngster candy or cookies while you are marketing; from that time on he will probably associate eating with shopping for groceries. On the occasions when begging for food becomes embarrassing or wears you down (where is that child psychologist who says children cannot concentrate on one subject?), a younger child can be given a slice of cheese or liverwurst or a hot dog of a reliable brand which you know has been precooked. A youngster of 3 years or older can be given these same foods or salted peanuts, popcorn, potato chips, or corn chips. Although the appetite for the next meal may be somewhat ruined, their thirst for milk will not be.

Skim milk versus whole milk for children. The cream on 1 quart of average milk supplies about 350 calories, 2,000 units of vitamin A, and, if the cows are kept on green food, a nutrient essential to growth known as vaccenic acid. Fats, however, satisfy the appetite more quickly and for a longer time than do proteins or carbohydrates. In case a child's appetite is poor, he should be given limited amounts of fat until his food intake has increased.

A diet high in protein is more health building than one rich in fat. If ½ cup of powdered skim milk is beaten into 1 quart of whole milk, the protein content is doubled, but the cream together with the increased protein may make the combined milks too satisfying. In this case the cream can be poured off the milk before the powdered milk is beaten into it. The child, however, should take the cream separately on cereal or sliced bananas or other food. Moreover, when skim milk is given instead of whole, a child can drink far more of it between meals without ruining his appetite for the next meal.

If the cream is removed over too long a period, the child may no longer enjoy the flavor of whole milk. Where the line should be drawn between giving whole milk for the nutrients of cream and giving skim milk to increase the intake of protein and calcium, each mother must decide for herself, depending on the needs of her child.

Bed wetting and milk intake. There seems to be general agreement that the causes of bed wetting are psychological, and that fears and muscular and nerve tensions are created by blame or overpraise or some faulty attitude on the part of the parents. I do not wish to imply in any way that drinking adequate amounts of milk can rectify such a situation. The frequently attempted remedy of cutting down liquids and thus decreasing the milk intake, however, can definitely make the problem worse.

Milk is the only food in our American diet from which adequate calcium can be obtained. Even a mild lack of calcium causes irritability and tension in nerves and muscles. When this cause of tension is added to the psychological causes, a child can have still less control of the muscles of his bladder. The practice of restricting all liquids after 4:00 P.M., therefore, is advisable only when the child has drunk 1 quart of milk earlier in the day. Even when bedding must be changed daily, the cost of laundering it is slight in comparison with the medical and dental bills which will probably arise if the milk intake is not kept adequate.

Drinking too much milk. Now and then one finds a child who practically lives on milk and eats little other food. Such a child is usually better off than the youngster who drinks too little, especially if yeast, blackstrap, and vitamin C are added. Such one-sidedness, however, can hardly be recommended. Milk alone is deficient in iron, some of the trace minerals, and vitamins C, D, and E; it supplies too little B vitamins to support ideal health.

If this problem arises, for a few days remove part or all of the cream (the most satisfying portion of the milk). A rule could be established that no milk would be allowed until other foods are eaten; the servings of these foods should be kept small, however, in order not to discourage the child. A generous amount of praise when other food is eaten usually works wonders. Unless the child's appetite for wholesome foods is being ruined by sweets, the problem of drinking milk and eating nothing else is usually of short duration and need not cause undue concern.

Milk is the most important food. It is often pointed out that many primitive people, Eskimos for example, stay healthy without drinking milk. Except during famines, the native Eskimo's diet is principally meat, which supplies him with ample protein and vitamin B_2; he eats fish bones from which he obtains adequate calcium. Various primitive races have other sources of these nutrients, but the sources are foods which no American would eat daily. Adequate diets can be planned which contain no milk, but it is extremely difficult for a child or even an adult to consume enough other foods to supply his requirements of protein, vitamin B_2, and calcium. In our American culture, there is no substitute for milk except milk in other forms such as buttermilk or yogurt.

Bear in mind, therefore, that throughout every year of your child's development milk is the most important food you can give him. Whenever certified raw milk is available, buy it for the family rather than any other. The extra cost will be compensated for by smaller medical and dental bills.

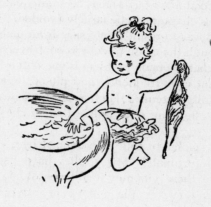

CHAPTER 18

HEALTH PROBLEMS DURING
INFANCY AND EARLY CHILDHOOD

W HEN both the mother's diet during pregnancy and the infant's food after birth have been adequate, the problems discussed in this chapter can be largely avoided. These deviations from health appear to result principally from malnutrition.

Colic. Although the cause of colic is controversial, most pediatricians agree that the main problem is one of gas in the intestinal tract. The infant cries frequently and piteously, and his tiny abdomen is painfully distended. He frequently passes gas by rectum, often with an offending odor unlike that of the normal infant's stool.

A condition similar to colic is produced by a diet deficient in B vitamins. Unfortunately few studies have been made of an undersupply of these vitamins in infants. When adults are put on such a diet, however, the number of enzymes produced by the stomach, pancreas, and intestines is markedly decreased. The contractions of the entire intestinal tract slow down so that food is not well mixed with digestive juices and enzymes; already digested food is not brought into contact with the absorbing surfaces of the intestinal walls where it can pass into the blood. Hence much food is incompletely digested and absorbed. Undigested food in the intestines supports the growth of millions of bacteria; during the bacterial breakdown of such food, quantities of gases are liberated; gas pain and flatulence result. These gases cause the stools to have an abnormal odor. In short, such a person suffers from "colic."

Since both breast milk and cows' milk are poor sources of the

B vitamins, and since the need for these vitamins is increased by the addition of the sweeter sugars to standard formulas, it is not surprising that a baby develops the same symptoms as those produced experimentally. Infants given adequate B vitamins from birth rarely if ever develop colic. Furthermore, colic usually disappears 2 or 3 days after these vitamins have been added to the formula.

As a safety measure, I usually recommend that tablets of digestive enzymes be given a colicky baby temporarily. Such tablets supplement the enzymes in the digestive tract until sufficient B vitamins can be absorbed to bring about normal digestion. Druggists usually carry a number of enzyme tablets capable of digesting proteins, fats, and sugars. A tablet can be wrapped in a piece of clean paper, crushed thoroughly with a hammer, and added to the formula just before it is given to the infant. If the enzymes were added in advance, they would digest the formula and bring about a marked change in flavor. Usually the enzyme preparation is needed for only 2 or 3 days; if sufficient B vitamins are given and the sugar in the formula is reduced in amount, or withdrawn, the condition is generally corrected by that time.

When the baby suffering from colic is being breast fed, a little yeast, blackstrap molasses, and a crushed enzyme tablet can be added to 1 ounce of juice or boiled water and given the baby after he has nursed a few minutes. It is important that the enzyme be in his digestive tract together with his food. In case of colic, the laxative effect of a little molasses is desirable; thus the waste material in the baby's bowel is forced out, and the amount of undigested food is so decreased that less gas can be formed.

If the infant's abdomen is distended with gas, and yet his stools do not have the offending odor which indicates bacterial fermentation, the problem may be one of merely too much swallowed air and inadequate burping. Air forced from the stomach into the intestine continues to expand as it heats to body temperature and can cause considerable pain. Rules given on page 150 should be observed, and crying from hunger should be avoided by the demand feeding and the use of pacifiers.

In the hospitals of Europe, yogurt [1] is often used in the treatment of infant colic and other digestive disturbances. The bacteria of yogurt live in the intestinal tract and break milk sugar (lactose) into lactic acid, which prevents the growth of gas-forming bacteria. Yogurt for infant feeding can be prepared by adding yogurt culture (p. 175) or 2 or 3 tablespoons of previously prepared yogurt to 1 quart of boiled and cooled whole or partially skim milk; it is kept at 110 degrees F. for 3 hours, or until it thickens. The yogurt is then thoroughly beaten so that it will pass through the nipple holes and is given to the baby instead of the usual formula. Vitamin C, yeast, and blackstrap may be added when the yogurt is beaten. Commercial yogurt can also be added to an infant's formula. If the baby is old enough to swallow easily, a thick yogurt can be given by spoon (p. 175).

Vomiting. Whenever vomiting becomes a problem, look for mechanical causes (p. 126). Make sure you are holding your baby in a sitting position as you feed him; do not allow him to become so hungry that he will gulp his meal; throw away old nipples, and buy a different type of bottle if necessary. Also see that your baby's diet contains a generous amount of the B vitamins. Vomiting has been produced experimentally in adults by diets deficient in vitamins B_1 or B_6. Furthermore, vomiting often ceases soon after all the B vitamins are given a baby.

Infants sometimes suffer from a condition spoken of as pyloristenosis, or spasm of the opening between the stomach and small intestine. This condition, characterized by the vomitus being expelled with such force that it may shoot from the mouth at a right angle to the body or in a wide arc, can be caused by a tumorlike growth. If it should develop, take your baby immediately to your pediatrician. Make sure, however, that the diet is adequate in the B vitamins. I have seen a number of cases clear up almost immediately when such foods as wheat germ, yeast, and liver or liver concentrate are given the infant.

Young mothers sometimes worry because the milk spit up when

[1] J. B. Mayer, "The Use of Yogurt in Feeding Infants Suffering from Intestinal Disturbances," *Nutrition Abs. and Rev.*, 3462, **18** (1949), 619.

a baby is burped is soured and curdled. The healthy stomach secretes hydrochloric acid, necessary for digestion. The first stage of the digestion of milk is curdling, which causes the milk to remain in the stomach long enough for enzymes to act upon it. Such soured, curdled milk, therefore, indicates only that your baby's digestion is quite normal.

Constipation. Constipation means a hard stool, not an infre-quent or small stool. The only harm of constipation is danger of mechanical injury to the anus. Many small children have only one bowel movement every other day and the movement is still soft and perfectly normal. I once took a course in infant feeding from the famous authority on child nutrition, Dr. Amy Daniels, in which she often remarked, "If a baby has only one bowel movement a month and the stool is still soft, the baby is not constipated."

Constipation can be readily overcome by giving an infant ade-quate amounts of the B vitamins in the form of brewers' yeast and/or blackstrap molasses. Even when the stools have been hard, no more than 1 teaspoon of blackstrap should be given the first day; later the amount can be decreased or gradually increased, depending on the texture of the stools the previous day. Black-strap molasses (1 or 2 teaspoons) daily together with 4 or 5 tea-spoons of brewers' yeast will certainly insure stools of soft texture.

Giving the baby too much butter fat can sometimes cause him to become constipated. If extremely rich milk is used for the formula, or if more fat is fed than is digested, the undigested fat can combine with the calcium of the milk to form a hard soap; the stools then have a shiny texture actually similar to soap in appearance. This form of constipation causes the baby to be robbed of valuable calcium. The remedy is to decrease the butter fat in the formula temporarily and to increase the B vitamins so that ample digestive enzymes can be produced to digest whatever fat is given.

The use of enemas. In the past, it has often been customary to give infants and small children enemas not only when they are constipated but also at the onset of a cold, a fever, or any sign of illness. It is probably correct to say that, under all circumstances, enemas do more harm than good. The equipment used in giving an enema is anything but sterile; the water is often dirty; bacteria thus introduced may result in an infection. The walls of the intestinal tract are made of tiny muscles, like small rubber bands; as water is introduced, some of these muscles may be broken, causing the muscle tone to be damaged.

Psychologists tell us that enemas are harmful and may lead to serious problems later. The infant and small child think of their excreta as being a part of themselves. To them, the forceful removing of the excreta appears much the same as the amputating of a finger or nose would to us. I recently heard a psychiatrist remark, "We are still having trouble with the pediatricians recommending enemas." In my opinion it is not the pediatricians but the grandmothers and older nurses and baby sitters who recommend enemas to young mothers desperate enough at the moment to follow any advice given them.

Color of stools. A few mothers, particularly young, inexperienced ones, sometimes become alarmed because the color of the stools differs from time to time. The color is largely determined by pigments secreted in the bile. These pigments, when exposed to oxygen, change from various shades of green to light yellow, tan, and brown. The color of the stools therefore varies, depending upon the amount of oxygen in the intestines and the length of time the food mass stays in the body. When food passes quickly through the intestinal tract, or when little oxygen is present, the color tends to be green. In case the passage is slower or much air has been swallowed, the pigments are changed by oxygen to yellow or tan. These colors are all perfectly normal, nothing to be worried about.

The color of certain foods, particularly beets and spinach, can often be seen in the stools, and mothers are likely to think that the baby is not digesting his food. Even if the food were totally undigested, some of the water-soluble vitamins, sugars, and certain minerals would dissolve out of the food as it soaks in the digestive juices. Although digestion may be incomplete, there is no cause for concern.

A young infant sometimes passes black, tarry stools. They indicate there has been bleeding in the intestinal tract. In case such stools are passed, see your pediatrician immediately.

Occasionally a mother will worry because she detects mucus in the stools. The intestinal walls secrete mucus, which serves to protect and lubricate them. Finding mucus in the stools, therefore, does not necessarily indicate an infection. If much mucus is passed, however, discuss the matter with your pediatrician.

Infant diarrheas. Diarrhea means liquid or unformed stools which stain the diapers but leave little or no residue. Strictly speaking, it does not mean stools which are unusually soft or frequent. Diarrhea can be caused by an intestinal infection, known as enteritis, which can be fatal. Babies 6 months old or older sometimes become infected with intestinal parasites which cause diarrhea. You should, therefore, consult your pediatrician immediately in case diarrhea occurs.

The principal reason for infant deaths a hundred years ago was diarrhea caused by dirty milk and unsterilized equipment. When an infant suffers from diarrhea, great care should be taken to see that all food, drinking water, bottles, and utensils used in preparing the formula are sterile.

One cause of diarrhea today appears to be the large amounts of sugar given to babies (ref. 3, p. 116). Dr. McCulloch of the Pediatrics Department of Washington University Medical School, set out to study the causes of noninfectious diarrhea in infants. He found that if formulas without added sugar were given, the stools were firmer in texture and decreased in number from an average of eight or ten daily to two or four daily. In all of the studies cited (pp. 116-119) of infants given formulas without added sugar, none suffered from diarrhea.

Another cause of diarrhea is lack of the B vitamin, niacin. Little niacin is found in either breast milk or cows' milk. This vitamin, however, can be produced in the body provided there is an ample supply of the amino acid, tryptophane, which a baby can obtain from the protein of milk. Since breast-fed babies receive less protein than do most bottle-fed infants, tiny babies who can take little milk obtain a meager supply of tryptophane, and little of the vitamin can be formed; hence breast-fed babies more frequently have a tendency to diarrhea than do artificially fed infants. When the formula is particularly low in protein, however, or when a baby can take only a small amount of food, little tryptophane is available, and diarrhea resulting from niacin deficiency may occur even in bottle-fed infants.

In any case of diarrhea, it is wise to give a formula high in protein and free from added sugar. The B vitamins should be supplied by the use of brewers' yeast, rich in niacin, starting with ¼ teaspoon per bottle and gradually increasing to 1 heaping teaspoon in each. Blackstrap molasses should be avoided. In cases of severe noninfectious diarrhea, pediatricians often recommended that a 50-milligram tablet of the pure vitamin, niacin amide, be given in each bottle of formula for 3 or 4 days. When the infant suffering from diarrhea is breast fed, both yeast and niacin amide should be taken by the mother as well as given to the infant in drinking water.

If your pediatrician recommends this vitamin to you, be particularly careful to get only the form niacin *amide;* niacin alone, although harmless, can cause flushing of skin, tingling, and itching and thus can make the baby uncomfortable and create a rather frightening experience for the mother.

When an infant suffers from diarrhea, most mothers believe that little food of any kind should be given; otherwise the diarrhea may become worse. A study was made at New York University Medical School of the feeding of infants who had severe diarrhea. The infants were given foods low, moderate, and high in calories. The amounts of minerals and of protein retained in the body were carefully checked. It was found that when small or moderate amounts of food were given, more nutrients were excreted than were retained. On the other hand, when the infants were allowed a high-calorie diet or were given as much food as they would eat, they absorbed and stored protein and minerals;

yet the diarrhea did not become worse. Some infants even gained weight in spite of severe diarrhea. The investigators found that if too little protein was given, water was held in the body, causing the babies to appear chubby and in good condition, whereas they were actually seriously ill. When the infants were given protein, the stored water was lost and their bodies were seen to be extremely thin.

A formula for an infant suffering from diarrhea, therefore, should be as concentrated as possible. If the baby is old enough to take solids, he should be allowed to eat as much high-protein food as he will take: eggs, cheese, thick yogurt (p. 175), meat, and only slightly sweetened custards and junkets. Such foods are nutritionally preferable to the baked potatoes, rice, and mashed banana customarily given for diarrhea.

Teething. Babies vary widely in their reaction to teething. One mother may have no idea a tooth is coming in until she discovers it, whereas another mother may be kept busy soothing an irritable and whining infant for days before she sees any signs of the tooth.

The healthy baby given a completely adequate diet usually suffers little when his teeth erupt. If the diet is inadequate, however, trouble can be expected. For example, a lack of vitamin C or of the B vitamin, niacin, causes the gums to be sore; such soreness is exaggerated by teething, and pain is undoubtedly intensified. It has been found that persons lacking certain B vitamins are more sensitive to pain than when these vitamins are adequate; probably the same reaction is experienced by infants. If a baby is given so little vitamin D that inadequate calcium is absorbed, he becomes irritable and restless, crying or whining much of the time; in such a case, teething makes him feel even more uncomfortable.

The diet, therefore, should be particularly adequate during the time the teeth are erupting. If your baby is especially irritable, it may be wise, for a few days, to increase the amounts of vitamins D and yeast slightly and of vitamin C considerably.

Just as the word allergy is used as a scapegoat to explain almost any obscure symptom, so is teething blamed for many abnormalities which occur during the time the teeth may be expected to erupt. Such abnormalities may indeed be caused by the teething. On the other hand, they may have no relation to it, but as long as teething is blamed, the real cause is not sought, nor is correction attempted. It is undoubtedly safest for your baby's health to assume that he will have no trouble teething. If he runs a temperature or becomes ill, see your pediatrician to make sure that the child is not suffering from an infection. The assumption that teething is responsible for upsets at this time has caused many babies to suffer serious illnesses which could have been alleviated if the pediatrician had seen the infant sooner.

Diaper rashes. Although there are many causes of diaper rashes, in my opinion such rashes occur principally when the child is undersupplied with vitamin A. If from birth a child is given plain halibut-liver oil or a concentrate of vitamin A in aqueous solution, in addition to some preparation supplying vitamin D, diaper rashes rarely occur. Quite severe rashes can usually be healed merely by giving 20 drops of halibut-liver oil after each feeding or 2 drops of vitamin A in aqueous solution in each bottle for a few days. Psychologists now stress that a baby's diapers should not be changed oftener than after each feeding unless the diaper is soiled or the infant has diaper rash. Even when the diapers are changed infrequently, no rash need result if the baby's diet is kept adequate.

What appears to be a diaper rash may be a mild form of eczema or an allergy. It may require further changes in the diet aside from increased vitamin A.

Other skin rashes. Many skin rashes occur which often disappear as readily as they have come. Heat rash is well known and can be corrected by dressing the baby less warmly. It is important for a mother to realize that a healthy full-term infant has a higher basal metabolism than does an adult. That is, he produces heat more efficiently and is therefore warmer than an older person. Many mothers have a tendency to keep their babies too warm, particularly if they themselves are below par and suffer from the cold.

When a rash appears, and its cause is unknown, it is well to increase vitamins A and C, the B vitamins, and particularly the unsaturated fatty acids (p. 101). To supply these acids, 3 or more teaspoons of corn or soybean oil should be given with each meal, either directly from a spoon or mixed with food. Only after such steps have been taken and the rash has not cleared up is the conclusion justified that the baby may be allergic to some food he is eating.

Nonallergic eczemas. Although eczemas are usually thought of as allergies, they frequently result from deficiencies of the B vitamins. A lack of any one of several B vitamins, such as vitamin B_2 (riboflavin), niacin, pantothenic acid, vitamin B_6 (pyridoxin), para aminobenzoic acid, and particularly biotin, results in skin abnormalities spoken of medically as dermatitis or by the layman as eczema.

Since the giving of one or more B vitamins appears to increase the need of any B vitamin not supplied, eczemas may be produced by giving babies certain multiple-vitamin preparations. Such preparations usually supply generous amounts of the cheaper synthetic B vitamins: B_1, B_2, B_6, niacin, and pantothenic acid; although the need for the lesser known B vitamins is thereby increased, they are not supplied. Multiple-vitamin preparations should certainly not be given to an infant suffering from eczema.

A baby with eczema should be given daily natural foods rich in all the known B vitamins. If yeast has not been given, it should be introduced at the rate of $\frac{1}{4}$ teaspoon per bottle. In case the baby is not old enough to eat solids, uncooked liver and wheat germ can be put into a blender (p. 177), mixed with milk and given from a bottle. For an older child, uncooked liver may be scraped with a spoon and served raw or heated slightly. Either raw or toasted wheat germ can be stirred into fruit or given as a cereal or mixed with whatever cereal is already being used. When these sources of B vitamins are fed, eczemas caused by such lack usually clear up rapidly.

Eczemas are often produced by giving babies raw or under-cooked egg white. A substance in raw egg white, avidin, combines with the B vitamin, biotin, and prevents it from reaching the blood; the resulting biotin deficiency causes the eczema. Only the yolk of hard-cooked eggs should be given to babies suffering from eczema. Since wheat germ, liver, and especially yeast are all rich in biotin, a deficiency of this vitamin can be prevented when these foods are included in the diet and eggs are properly prepared.

Sometimes eczemas in infants are caused by a lack of unsaturated fatty acids, found in the oils of corn, soybeans, and wheat germ. Any of these oils can be put directly into an infant's mouth by a dropper or spoon.

Colds. It is doubtful whether even the best diet can keep a child entirely free from colds. The most important factor in preventing colds appears to be isolation, or avoiding contact with anyone suffering from a cold, particularly during its early stages. It has been found, however, that when the nutrition is inadequate, colds occur more frequently, are more severe, and hang on for longer periods than when the diet is excellent.

A treatment now recommended for adults coming down with a cold is to take ten 100-milligram tablets of vitamin C as soon as the first symptoms appear; then to take three to five 100-milligram tablets every 3 hours until the cold is gone. A number of mothers I know have used a variation of this treatment whenever their infants appear to be getting colds; they claim to have met with marked success. They have given five or six tablets of vitamin C, 100 milligrams each, melted in 1 ounce of boiling water and sweetened to taste or added to a sweet juice as soon as the onset of a cold was noticed; in the same manner they gave 200 or 300 milligrams more of the vitamin every few hours. If the symptoms are not severe, the extra vitamin C can be added to the formula.

If the diet of a healthy baby or child is adequate in vitamin C, much of this vitamin is lost in the urine when more than 50 milligrams are given at one time. In case of colds, however, large amounts are given without any being lost in the urine. Vitamin C, or ascorbic acid, serves as a detoxifying mechanism in the body. It appears to combine with virus or any foreign substance, and the combination of the vitamin and the foreign material, spoken of as ascorbigen, is then excreted in the urine. For this reason, large quantities of the vitamin are needed at the onset of a cold or other infection and for the duration of the illness; hence they can be taken at such times without urinary loss. Since any of the vitamin not needed is thrown off in the urine, massive doses are not harmful; therefore it is better to err by giving too much than too little.

Whenever colds occur frequently or hang on a long time, a deficiency of vitamin A can be suspected. Such a deficiency can be prevented by giving an infant some preparation rich in vitamin A in addition to his regular cod-liver oil or other source of vitamin D; 20 drops or more of plain halibut-liver oil daily or 6 to 10 drops of vitamin A in aqueous solution (p. 94) might be used. During a cold, it is probably wise to give the vitamin-A preparation with each feeding or afterward.

Bronchitis, pneumonia, and other infections. Much the same procedure as recommended for colds should be followed when a baby has bronchitis, pneumonia, or any other infection involving mucous membranes, such as infections of the sinuses, middle ears, or kidneys. Frequently a mother becomes frightened and stops the vitamins recommended by her pediatrician at the very time they are most needed; thus the more ill the child, the more inadequate his nutrition becomes. Increased amounts of vitamins A and C should be continued for the duration of the infection even though it may last for weeks.

In order to prevent infections, it is particularly important that the baby's formula and other food be rich in protein. The principal mechanisms for fighting infections are antibodies, white blood cells, and similar cells throughout the body, known as phagocytes. These cells cannot be produced by the body unless the protein intake is adequate. Experiments have shown that when a diet is changed from one low in protein to one rich in protein, antibody production is increased a hundredfold within a week's time.

Importance of frequent feedings during illness. When a baby or child becomes so ill that his appetite is poor, the first thing to do is to give him small, frequent feedings of some food which contains natural sugar. If no food or very little food is eaten for several hours, a condition known as acetone acidosis occurs. This condition is caused by the amount of sugar in the blood dropping below normal; it is common even among well children who fail to eat enough or who obtain too little protein.

Acidosis can be detected on the breath, which gives off an odor of acetone. If you are not familiar with acetone, which is used to remove nail polish, buy some polish remover or ask a druggist to allow you to smell acetone. Every mother should recognize this odor in order to identify acidosis.

Whenever acetone acidosis occurs, the baby or child becomes irritable and restless, cries readily and frequently vomits. If no sugar or sugar-forming food is eaten, the vomiting may become so severe that the child must be hospitalized and given glucose injections. The mother, who may never have heard of acidosis, naturally assumes that the illness has caused the vomiting and makes no effort to increase the blood sugar. In all probability, the vomiting which accompanies most childhood illnesses and diseases is brought about because the child feels too ill to eat.

It is wise to give an ill baby or child a small amount of food every 1 or 2 hours: 1 ounce or more of orange, pineapple, grape, apple, or other sweet juice or sweetened lemonade; ½ teaspoon of honey or molasses; or a cracker for an older child. It has been found that vitamin C detoxifies acetone; hence 1 teaspoon or more of vitamin-C solution (p. 132) should be added to any liquid for the child. If he refuses all food, the vitamin C should be sweetened and given alone. A small amount of sugar, preferably milk sugar, may be added to a baby's formula until the appetite is again normal. If a little food is taken frequently enough, vomiting can be prevented. In case a strong odor of acetone can be detected or the child is already vomiting, the frequent feedings become still more important; they should be offered every hour, even though you may expect most of the food to be thrown up again. Some of it will eventually be retained and the condition corrected. The frequent feedings should be continued until the breath is sweet again.

Probably every mother has had to deal with acetone acidosis. A mother recently called me to say that her 2-year-old boy had been ill the day before; he now appeared to feel better but was vomiting frequently. When I asked her to smell his breath, she reported that it had an odd odor. She then gave him pineapple juice with vitamin C every hour; although he threw up most of two feedings, he did not vomit after that. When a mother is aware that acetone acidosis occurs and when she tries to prevent vomiting, it rarely becomes a severe problem.

Leave the drugs to your pediatrician. No mother should give a baby or child drugs, regardless of how valuable they may be in the hands of a physician. For example, a pediatrician may recommend one of the barbiturates for a baby suffering from colic, intending that it be given for only 2 or 3 days. The mother, understandably grateful for a few nights of uninterrupted sleep, may get the prescription refilled and continue giving the drug for weeks or even months. Aside from the fact that nothing constructive is being done to improve the infant's health, barbiturates are detoxified by vitamin C and can cause the baby to develop a severe deficiency of this vitamin even though it may be generously supplied in the diet. The induced deficiency of vitamin C, in turn, can inhibit normal growth and dental development; it may cause the child to become susceptible to allergies and infections. Thus it may do far more harm than the barbiturate could possibly do good.

Similarly the giving of aspirin and related compounds known as salicylates can bring about a deficiency not only of vitamin C but, if given over a long period or in large quantities, of vitamin K [2,3] as well. It is conceivable that an accident might occur after a mother has given her child too much aspirin and that bleeding

---

[2] "Salicylates and Hemorrhages," *Lancet,* 2 (1943), 2, 419.

[3] Editorial: "Is Aspirin a Dangerous Drug?" *J. Am. Med. Assn.,* 124 (1944), 777.

could be fatal, whereas it might have been insignificant if vitamin K had not been destroyed. Since it is now known that vitamin C acts as a detoxifying mechanism and is needed in large quantities during colds or any infections, the giving of aspirin at such times seems particularly unwise.

The sulfa drugs, known collectively as sulfonamides, and such drugs as penicillin, streptomycin, aureomycin, and chloromycetin, known as the antibiotics, have been found to produce deficiencies of vitamins C and K and several of the B vitamins. Studies have been made of the amount of vitamins in the blood before and after these drugs have been given. Although the diet remained exactly the same after the drugs had been given, the amount of vitamins C and K and the B vitamins decreased to that of marked deficiency and remained deficient over long periods. The body's supply of vitamin C is apparently used to detoxify the drug, whereas the drug itself destroys the valuable bacteria of the intestinal tract, thus preventing the synthesis of vitamin K and the B vitamins. Yet I know of a number of mothers who have prescriptions of these drugs refilled time and again. Without consulting a pediatrician, they give the drugs to their babies or small children at the first sign of a sniffle.

A recent report [4] indicates that the destruction of valuable bacteria in the intestines by the use of drugs may have serious and lasting effects. An infection known to the layman as thrush and caused by a fungus, Monilia albicans, which normally inhabits the bowel, may overgrow and perhaps become virulent following the destruction of valuable intestinal bacteria. This infection may invade tissues the resistance of which has been lowered by deficiency of vitamin B_2 and other B vitamins which is also produced by the drug. A physician with whom I discussed this report told me that he found thrush in almost every case where penicillin or aureomycin or a similar drug had been given over a period of 10 days; although thrush could be

4 H. J. Harris, "Aureomycin and Chloramphenical (Chloromycetin) in Brucellosis with Special Reference to Side Effects," *J. Am. Med. Assn.*, 142 (1950), 161.

prevented easily, it was extremely difficult to clear up after it has once gained a foothold. He further stated that whenever he finds it necessary to use a sulfonamide or an antibiotic, he first makes sure that the patient's intake of the B vitamins is doubled or tripled, and he advises that yogurt be eaten daily for several weeks to replace intestinal bacteria.

It would undoubtedly be wise to follow this doctor's suggestions as to diet in case your pediatrician finds it necessary to give a similar drug to your child. Whenever any drug must be given, however, increase the amount of vitamin C in his formula or diet. The quantities of vitamin C, yogurt, and foods supplying the B vitamins would vary with the amount of the drug administered; it is probably advisable to give as much as the child will take.

A drug, wisely used by a competent pediatrician, may save your child's life; that same drug, unwisely used by a mother, may seriously interfere with his health.

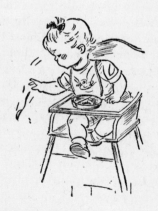

CHAPTER 19

YOUR CHILD HAS THE RIGHT
TO BE BEAUTIFUL

I BELIEVE that you, as a mother, will largely determine whether or not your child will be beautiful. I believe that the factors which determine beauty more than any others are the nutrients necessary for the development of normal bones. If these nutrients are generously supplied from birth *throughout the entire growth period,* the chances are that your girls will be beautiful and your sons handsome. If the nutrients are not adequately supplied, the chances are small indeed.

Probably every nutrient plays some role, directly or indirectly, in the building of normal bones and teeth. Skeletal development can be retarded or even cease temporarily because of the lack of any one of four nutrients: vitamins C and D, protein, and calcium. Phosphorus is equally important, but it is so generously supplied in foods that it is rarely if ever lacking in the diet.

Most mothers, aware of the importance of calcium, make every effort to see that their children drink enough milk to supply this mineral. If the child eats so little protein, however, that none can be stored in the body (negative nitrogen balance), all the calcium obtained and more will be lost in the urine and feces.[1] The new cells which form the base of the bones and are made of protein, cannot develop unless adequate protein is supplied; without these cells, calcium cannot be laid down. Vitamin C is also necessary in the formation of the base of teeth and bones; it gives strength to both and elasticity to the bones. If

[1] J. A. Johnson, "The Calcium and Vitamin D Requirements of the Older Child," *Am. J. Dis. Child.,* **67** (1944), 265.

a deficiency of this vitamin should occur, the calcium obtained in food is lost in the urine and feces, and cells already formed in the teeth and bones break down, freeing minerals which are likewise excreted. Without vitamin D, neither calcium nor phosphorus is efficiently absorbed or utilized normally in building skeletal structure.

Most babies get some vitamin C from orange juice and obtain protein and calcium from milk. The limiting factor during babyhood, therefore, is most often a lack of vitamin D. So little vitamin D occurs in foods that for all practical purposes it is correct to say that foods lack it. The only sources of this vitamin worth mentioning are fish-liver oils, fish-liver-oil concentrates, foods to which the vitamin has been added, sunshine, oils irradiated by ultraviolet light, and special preparations such as viosterol or vitamin D in aqueous solution.

If your baby is to be beautiful, he must be given vitamin D. The bone abnormalities which occur when a baby is undersupplied with vitamin D are spoken of as rickets. This disease was almost universal a few years ago.

My first job after I had finished dietetics training was at the Judson Health Center in lower New York City. The people who came to the Health Center were largely Italians who had emigrated from Southern Italy and Sicily. Baby clinics were held several times each week. The three of us who worked as nutritionists were instructed to listen to the physician's diagnosis and then to tell the mother how to feed her baby, the points to stress depending upon the diagnosis. The diagnoses, however, were at least in part almost always the same: rickets, rickets, rickets.

There were times when we were too busy talking to mothers to hear the doctor's diagnosis; hence the several fine pediatricians who gave their time to the clinic trained us to recognize poor bone structure. The instructions were somewhat like this: "Look at the baby's profile; the forehead should be flat and straight with the general line of the face, not rounded or bulging outward. As you look directly into the infant's face, the bones above the ears should be a straight line with the cheekbones below; they should not flare outward. There should be width of bone between the eyes and from the outer edges of the eyes to the ears. The eyes should not be set too deeply in the head or be crowded together. When the baby is lying flat, before the mother dresses him, look closely at the chest; it should be broad and rounded and almost barrel-shaped, like the chests of most infants when they are born. The chest should not be narrow or flat between the shoulders, and the lower ribs should not flare out or upward. When the child is held in a standing position, the stomach should not be large and bulging nor should the chest bone, or sterum, be raised into a pigeon chest." There were other instructions about straight legs and normally developed wrist bones. After months of such training we no longer saw dimples and long eyelashes but only bone structure.

To each mother we stressed the importance of giving the baby cod-liver oil or cod-liver-oil concentrate every day and of taking him to the roof for sunbaths. But cod-liver oil cost money and made the baby smell bad; and to reach the tenement roof the mothers had to climb perhaps six flights of stairs through halls as dark as midnight even on the sunniest days. (When we made home calls, we carried flashlights with us.) Besides, no one ever heard of giving babies cod-liver oil in Italy, and they grew all right.

Some of the mothers, however, gave the oil conscientiously, and we watched the bulging foreheads and flared ribs gradually change to normal; their babies became beautiful children. Other mothers gave the oil part of the time, when they remembered it or could afford it. The enlargements of their babies' bones disappeared, but the skeletal structure remained underdeveloped. The little faces stayed narrow, perhaps with receding jaws and slanting foreheads, the eyes too close together, and the chests hollow and underdeveloped. These children were not pretty, and their bone structure showed slight resemblance to that of their parents. Other mothers gave neither cod-liver oil nor sunbaths, and their babies grew to be ugly, misshapen children. Yet most of these babies were nursed, and the mothers rarely failed to give them orange juice, a food which they themselves enjoyed. It was vitamin D or lack of it which determined whether their children were beautiful or ugly.

Some babies, mostly ill or premature ones, can drink so little milk that they do not receive enough calcium and protein to build normal bones. Others are given formulas so diluted with water that they cannot drink enough to supply the nutrients needed. In other cases, sugars which interfere with calcium absorption are added to the formula in such quantities that the minerals cannot pass into the blood. In any of these cases, rickets may occur, even though vitamin D is supplied.

Stop blaming your relatives. Whenever I point out to a mother that her child's bone structure is not perfect, the reply is invariably, "He looks exactly like his father." Or perhaps it is Uncle Henry or grandmother or some other relative. Although family resemblances are inherited, faulty bone structure is not. It is just as easy to allow your child to be a beautiful miniature of his father or Uncle Henry or grandmother as to be an ugly one. Poor bone structure should not be accepted as inevitable regardless of how similar it is to that of another relative. The chances are that the diets father and Uncle Henry and grandmother ate during their own childhood were inadequate in many nutrients.

More than any other person, the late Dr. Weston A. Price showed that abnormal bone structure could not be inherited. Dr. Price studied primitive peoples throughout the world and the effect of their diets upon their dental and bone structure. He found that when they ate their native diets, which were amazingly adequate because no refined foods could be obtained, certain characteristics were evident: their facial bones were broad, their eyes widely spaced, and their cheekbones well developed; the lower third of their faces was wide, and the jawbones were sufficiently large to permit the teeth to be even and straight without crowding; their chins were strong and broad and in no case receding.

Dr. Price also found people of the same races who had adopted the worst features of a white man's diet, chiefly foods which can be shipped without spoiling: white-flour products, refined sugar, canned foods, and coffee. Children raised on such a diet were different indeed from their parents who had lived on native foods. Almost every type of skeletal malformation could be found: narrow, "shallow" faces; thin, elongated foreheads; eyes crowded together; almost a hollowness under the eyes and through the cheekbones. The distance between the ears was proportionately perhaps a third less than that of the parents. Furthermore, almost 100 per cent of these children had narrow jaws and crooked, crowded teeth. Pictures of these people can be seen in Dr. Price's excellent book, *Nutrition and Physical Degeneration;* and his slides which are available to everyone.[*] Most striking to me was the underdevelopment of the bones through the middle third of the face; when looked at in profile, such a face could be described as having a shallowness or an inward curve instead of an outward one, causing the person with such a bone formation to appear stupid.

In a few instances, Dr. Price found families of three living generations where the grandparents had grown up on native foods, and the parents had lived in a white man's settlement and been raised on an inferior diet, but before having their children they had returned to remote spots where only natural food was again available. The bone structure of these third-generation children resembled that of their grandparents, not that of their parents. Their entire skeletal structure was beautifully developed.

The abnormalities of bone structure similar to those found by Dr. Price exist in America in millions of faces. Unfortunately most of us need to look no farther than into a mirror to see them. Many infants are born with abnormal bone structure; when a mother's diet during pregnancy is inadequate, normal bones cannot be formed. Such abnormalities, though congenital, should not be considered hereditary even when a parent has similar faulty

[*] The book and slides can be obtained from the American Academy of Applied Nutrition, 1105 S. LaBrea Ave., Los Angeles, California.

bone structure. Hundreds of other children, perfect at birth, are growing up with poor skeletal development because they have received inadequate diets; both groups could become beautiful children if the value of nutrition were more fully appreciated and if relatives were not blamed for unattractive family resemblances.

Instead of the usual attitude, I once heard a more intelligent point of view expressed. A man and wife who by their own admission are not especially attractive have one of the most beautiful little girls I have ever seen. The mother remarked to me, "We often wonder which one of us might have looked like her if we had been raised on a good diet."

Variations in faulty bone structure. Although a baby may be born with poor skeletal development, defects are usually first noticeable at about the fifth or sixth month. If no vitamin D has been given, or if calcium has been undersupplied or poorly absorbed for any reason, certain bones become enlarged: the breastbone, or sterum, the lower ribs and the ends of the arm bones at the wrists and leg bones at the knees. The most obvious abnormality is the enlargement of the head and forehead, causing the bones to flare out above the ears and eyes. The cartilagelike base of the bones becomes abnormally thick, as if nature were attempting to compensate for the lack of minerals and give strength or protection where either is most needed. Such an infant is usually irritable and restless; he cries and perspires easily. His teeth are late in erupting. When the child starts to walk, certain bones may bend, principally those of the legs, forming bowlegs, and those of the vertebrae, causing lordosis, or sway-back. If the diet is improved and sufficient vitamin D is given, the bones gradually become normal again; otherwise the skeletal abnormalities are carried throughout life, causing ugliness and unhappiness which could have been prevented.

Since almost every mother now gives her baby sunbaths and/or some form of vitamin D, severe cases of rickets are infrequently seen today. The abnormalities common now are in the form of underdevelopment of the bones which occurs when the diet is faulty or too little vitamin D is given. The face of a child whose diet has been inadequate in the bone-forming nutrients may show one or more of the following characteristics: narrowness, with perhaps receding forehead or chin; shallowness through the cheekbones; a pinched look across the eyes; or underdeveloped jawbones, causing the teeth to be crowded or crooked; flat, narrow chest; flared or underdeveloped lower ribs.

Actually every variation or combination of variations occurs, depending upon the inadequacy of the nutrients needed to build bones. A child may have a flared or overhanging forehead and underdeveloped middle and lower thirds of the face; such a child has the appearance of a thug selected for the movies. Perhaps only the lower third of the face is normal, the upper two-thirds being underdeveloped; by contrast the mouth seems to protrude into a "horse face"; or he may have an enlarged forehead and an underdeveloped jaw, which make him appear weak in character. Such bone structure is not spoken of as rickets but merely as faulty skeletal growth.

If a child whose bones have not developed as they should is given an adequate diet, the bones resume normal growth. His forehead will become straight and wide, the eyes may become farther apart, and his chin and cheekbones will develop normally. Such a child becomes immeasurably more attractive than one whose bone development is faulty.

Straight teeth add to attractiveness. Whenever the jawbones are underdeveloped, the teeth must necessarily be crowded together; hence they are usually crooked. On the other hand, if a child is given a diet adequate in all bone-building nutrients and absorbs them efficiently, even though his jawbones are small and his teeth already crowded together, the jawbones will grow and allow the teeth to fall into line as even as piano keys. Actually, when space allows, the teeth are pushed into line by the tongue and are held there by the pressure of the cheeks and lips except in cases where thumb sucking or mouth breathing may exert greater pressure.

One of the best ways for a mother to judge the adequacy of the diet she is giving her children is to observe their teeth and jawbones. The ideal dental arch, or the jawbone holding the teeth, should be almost a perfect semicircle; there is plenty of room in such a mouth for all the teeth without crowding. The dental arch should not be the shape of a tall U and certainly not V-shaped, as many are. The roof of the mouth, or dental vault, should be low and rounded like the roof of a Quonset hut, not like that of a high Swiss chalet built so that snows slide off quickly.

Look at your baby's mouth the day he is born and watch it throughout the entire growth period. If the arch is not semicircular or if the vault is high, see that the diet is especially adequate in all respects and that vitamin D is generously supplied. In time the jawbones will widen, and a V-shaped dental arch will gradually become U-shaped, or a U-shaped one become more and more semicircular. The roof of the mouth will simultaneously become lower and more rounded. The teeth, if crooked, will gradually fall into line provided the diet meets the needs of the child.

How extensive is faulty bone structure? A few years ago a study was made of the bone development of children in two cities: San Diego, California; and Portland, Oregon. The purpose was to find how effective sunshine was in preventing or correcting abnormal bone structure. San Diego was selected as having more hours of sunshine than any other city in the United States, and Portland as representative of cities having an average amount. In both cities several hundred children under 5 years old were carefully examined and their bones x-rayed, and no child was pronounced to have rickets unless he showed four or more signs of the disease. It was found that 95 per cent of all the children examined in Portland and 73 per cent of those examined in San Diego had rickets. A still more disconcerting fact was that 82 per cent of all the children had been given some form of cod-liver oil.

To anyone interested in children's health, let alone attractiveness, such findings are startling. A dozen questions arise. What is wrong with sunshine that almost three-fourths of these San Diego children had abnormal bone structure? If 82 per cent of the children were given some form of cod-liver oil, why were the bone abnormalities not prevented or cured by the oil? Since most babies are taken to private pediatricians or to clinics, why did not the doctors see that enough vitamin D was given to build normal bones? Let us try to find answers to these questions.

Why sunshine may not be a dependable source of vitamin D. For years it has been taught that the ultraviolet rays of the sun change a fatlike substance (ergosterol) in the skin into vitamin D; that the vitamin is also formed in the skin when it is exposed to the ultraviolet rays from lamps. Such information can be found in books on vitamins published only this year. It appears, however, that vitamin D is formed not *in* the skin but *on* the skin, which from a practical point of view makes all the difference in the world.

Studies made by Helmer and Jansen [2] have shown that the oil washed from the bodies of athletes after they have been exposed to ultraviolet light contains vitamin D. On the other hand, if the athletes were not exposed to sunshine or ultraviolet light, the oil contained no vitamin D. In this research, the body oil was washed off even with clear water, presumably cold, but more was removed when soap was used. When the oil containing the vitamin was rubbed on the skin of rachitis rats, enough was absorbed to cure the disease provided it was not washed off too soon. Heretofore the effect of bathing on human beings has been almost completely overlooked, largely because research is done with animals which do not bathe daily, nor do they hear or read hundreds of soap advertisements.

It has been suspected for many years that vitamin D is formed *on* the skin of animals and then absorbed through the skin or eaten or licked off. For example, if rachitic rats are washed daily, or if they are prevented from licking their fur, the disease is not cured by sunshine or ultraviolet light. It is known that show horses which are frequently washed develop rickets; that when

[2] A. C. Helmer and C. H. Jansen, "The Absorption of Vitamin D Through the Skin," and "Vitamin D Precursors Removed from Human Skin by Washing," *Studies of the Institutum Divi Thomae*, 1 (1937), 83, 207.

animals in zoos are given only the flesh of their prey without fur or feathers, they too develop the disease. For example, an owl becomes rachitic if not given the fur of mice, which contains vitamin D. Chickens develop rickets if their oil glands (preen glands) are removed. When a fowl preens itself, it spreads oil over its feathers, and the vitamin D formed by the sunlight is absorbed through the skin or eaten off. In all probability cats and rabbits lick their fur in order to obtain vitamin D rather than merely to cleanse themselves, and it has been suggested (ref. 2, p. 39) that a monkey's search for fleas is really his means of obtaining the vitamin.

One of the old wives' tales is that bathing a baby too much made him restless. Since no fish-liver oil was formerly given to babies, bathing probably washed off their only source of vitamin D, formed by chance exposure to sunshine; and rickets, characterized by restlessness, developed.

Medical and nutrition textbooks contain many pictures of children with severe rickets and the same children after they were cured by repeated exposures to sunlight. These pictures were largely taken by Dr. Chick [3] and her associates, who went to Vienna following the first world war to see whether rickets in humans could be cured by sunshine as it could in experimental animals. The fact that fuel was scarce and hot water and soap were even scarcer was overlooked. The chances are that the children cured by sunlight were not bathed as frequently or as soapily as were the children in the San Diego-Portland study or as are your children or mine.

During the last 4 years I have watched two little girls who live at the beach, neighbors of friends of mine. These children are as brown as coconuts both winter and summer. They have, however, all the classical signs of rickets, and their bone structure has not improved as they have grown older. The mother keeps the youngsters spotlessly clean. I suspect their only source of vitamin D is being scrubbed off.

[3] H. Chick et al., "Studies of Rickets in Vienna, 1919-1922," *Medical Research Council, Special Report Series,* No. 77, London, 1923.

You can find endless examples of faulty skeletal structure among children coming from our better homes. If you go into the poorer section of almost any city—the Mexican section of Los Angeles, for example—you can see many children who have beautiful bone structure. You can find similar children in farming communities where indoor plumbing is uncommon, and the Saturday-night bath may still be an honored institution. I suspect the difference lies neither in the quantity of milk, orange juice, and fish-liver oil consumed nor in the amount of sunshine obtained, but in the number of hot-water heaters and the amount of soap used. The beautiful skeletal development of the early American Indians and of many other primitive peoples was probably due, in part at least, to their lack of soap and hot water.

If vitamin D is to be obtained from sunshine, it is probably wise to bathe with cool or lukewarm rather than hot water and to use soap only when necessary. Bathing should be avoided immediately before exposure to sunshine so that the oil will not be removed, and immediately after exposure so that vitamin D will not be lost. It is not known how long one should wait for maximum absorption of the vitamin. It may help to put a thin layer of a vegetable oil on the skin before sunbathing. Allow your children to play in the sunshine as much as possible and to receive all the value they can from it. Since we certainly will continue to bathe and to use soap, however, it seems to me that the time has come for most of us to stop relying on sunshine as the only source of vitamin D.

Bone abnormalities can develop when cod-liver oil is given. Why did 82 per cent of the children in the San Diego-Portland study develop poor bone structure though they had been given some form of cod-liver oil? There are many reasons; sometimes all of them apply to the same child. Often the amount of vitamin D given is too small. The vitamin may be given hit or miss: it is easily forgotten, and it costs money. It is rarely continued over a sufficiently long period; bones may grow normally until the child is 1 or 2 years old and then become abnormal whenever vitamin D is stopped. Often a vitamin-D concentrate in oil is put directly into the bottles; although the coating cannot be seen, it adheres to the glass and nipples and the baby gets little or none of the vitamin. The most frequent mistake, however, lies in giving vitamin D in oil at a time when it cannot be absorbed into the blood.

Vitamin D in oil is carried across the intestinal wall into the blood only after it has combined with bile salts. Bile flows into the intestine after food is eaten. Yet many books on infant feeding and even government bulletins advise mothers to give the oil before the baby's bath but not to feed him until after his bath; the mothers are thus actually told to give the oil at a time when the vitamins in it cannot be properly absorbed. When vitamin D is given in aqueous solution (p. 94), this problem does not arise.

Another reason for faulty skeletal development is that no amount of vitamin D can compensate for a lack of other nutrients needed for bone growth. If the baby's bottle is taken away from him against his will, he may get too little calcium, phosphorus, and protein to build normal bones. Vitamin C may also be undersupplied. Often an older child receives vitamin C irregularly and drinks so little milk that he obtains less calcium from his food than is excreted; his protein may likewise be inadequate. Such a child will not have normal bones regardless of how much vitamin D is given him.

Faulty bone structure is usually not recognized. Let us go to our third question: since most children are taken to pediatricians or to well-baby clinics, why can rickets not be completely prevented or corrected? It was formerly believed that rickets was a condition which developed during the first year, and that if the bones grew satisfactorily at that period, they would continue to develop along normal lines. Now it is recognized that a child can have excellent skeletal structure as long as the diet remains adequate, but if deficiencies in the bone-building nutrients occur at any time during the growth period, the bones can become abnormal with amazing speed. Since many of the children in the San Diego-Portland study were 5 years old, it may be that most of them had excellent bone structure when they were 1 year old and under the supervision of physicians. After this age pediatricians rarely see children at regular intervals; the vitamin D is usually stopped, the diet becomes generally inadequate, and bone abnormalities start to appear.

Not long ago at a swimming pool I saw a 3-year-old girl whom I had not seen since she had learned to walk. She had been a beautiful baby; her little face had been round and her body sturdily built. Her face is now narrow and long and has a "pinched" look across the eyes; her teeth are crooked and crowded together; her chest is flat and caved in, the lower ribs flaring over a protruding stomach. Her mother remarked that she was ashamed to have the girl seen in a bathing suit. Even though the faulty bone structure was obvious, the mother had no idea why the change had come about. She did not even plan to take the child to a physician to find out how to correct the skeletal faults.

One reason such a large percentage of the children studied in San Diego and Portland were found to have faulty bone structure was that the doctors making the study were looking for abnormalities in skeletal development. Abnormalities common now are not easily noticed unless a person looks for them. The pediatricians have been most conscientious in recommending sunbaths and fish-liver oils or other preparations of vitamin D and in checking the mothers to make sure that these recommendations are followed. On the other hand, the doctors have been told many times during their training that bone abnormalities are prevented by sunshine or vitamin-D preparations; consequently when a mother assures them that her child is getting both, it may not occur to them to look for bone abnormalities.

The relation of skeletal development to dental health. Well-formed teeth, free from decay, add no small part to attractiveness. Since the nutrients necessary to build bones are needed for dental development, excellent bone structure and well-formed teeth, resistant to decay, are usually found together. When the diet is adequate in bone-building nutrients, the enamel of the teeth is thick, densely calcified, and free from pits and fissures; the dentine is likewise thick and almost as hard as the enamel itself. Although the main cause of decay appears to be the chewing of gum and the eating of too many sweets, such teeth are resistant to decay.

If any nutrient necessary for normal skeletal development is undersupplied or lacking during the years when the teeth are forming, the enamel can be thin, full of pits and fissures, and poorly calcified; the dentine may be so poorly mineralized that under a microscope it appears to have the texture of honeycomb. Such teeth decay rapidly. Animal experiments have shown that teeth which have been well calcified can quickly become honeycombed whenever the diet is inadequate. Fortunately, however, experiments in which radioactive minerals have been fed have proved that when the diet is adequate again, even at any time during the entire growth period, calcium and phosphorus can be laid down in both the dentine and the enamel; thus faulty tooth structure can be rectified. Mothers are sometimes inclined to excuse their children's tooth decay by saying that their own diets during pregnancy had been inadequate; thus they imply that nothing can be done to prevent further decay. The diet during pregnancy is important but principally in the formation of the baby teeth.

A year ago a mother asked me to check the diet of her two little girls because of rampant tooth decay. The mother had taken no form of vitamin D during pregnancy and had drunk little milk. She said that as infants both children had had flared ribs and bulging foreheads. The mother had given them 4 drops of cod-liver-oil concentrate daily for a time but only *before* feedings. She had stopped it when they were a few months old because of the expense and because no one told her it was important. The children's teeth were late in erupting and were crooked with relation to the jaws, warnings that the nutrients needed for skeletal development were being undersupplied. Active decay started when the children were 3 years old and had continued since. The older child had had nineteen new cavities at one time; both had had a series of dental abscesses and gumboils. One child's collar bone had broken twice when she had fallen out of swings, and a wrist bone had been shattered; the other had suffered a broken arm from tumbling on the grass. The mother had kept records of her dental bills; she had spent a total of $617 in 4 years, $213 in 1 year alone.

The daily diet I recommended was simple enough: a quart of raw certified milk with ½ cup of powdered milk added; 8 ounces of fresh orange juice; wheat germ to be used in cooking; 2 calcium tablets to be taken before breakfast and dinner; 1 vitamin-A capsule after breakfast. A capsule supplying 25,000 units of vitamin D was to be taken twice each week for a while, then after breakfast every Sunday. The children had avoided all forms of refined sugar and white flour for more than 2 years.

During the past year, one child has had a single cavity, compared with thirteen the year before, whereas the other has had none. The latter did, however, have an old filling replaced. Their dentist told me that formerly the dentine had been soft and crumbly but that it was now so hard that it was most difficult to drill into it.

In all probability, the structure of any child's teeth could be similarly improved if his diet were kept adequate.

Other advantages of normal bone structure. Aside from attractiveness, normal bone structure offers other advantages. When the skull is well formed, the sinuses, or holes in the face bones, are large; the thin mucus which continually bathes the membranes lining the sinuses can readily drain into the throat. If the bones of the face are small and poorly developed, the sinuses are particularly susceptible to infection, and pus often drains slowly from them, backing up to cause pressure face-aches and headaches. It is said that well-developed sinuses are necessary to give a pleasant resonance to the voice and that only persons with such sinuses can become great singers. The fact that many opera singers formerly came from Italy may be related to the abundance of sunshine, the scarcity of hot-water heaters, and a moderate use of soap.

Persons with underdeveloped chests are susceptible to respira-

tory infections. Adenoids sometimes become a problem partly
because the bones behind the nose are not spaced widely enough
apart to allow even slightly enlarged adenoids enough room.
When the bones of the shoulders, vertebrae, or pelvis are poorly
formed, backaches may occur and have to be endured for years.
Underdeveloped pelvic bones in women often necessitate Caesarean sections when they have their children. Subtle but still
abnormal bone development in the back, legs, and feet is one
reason why people run their shoes over on one side and may
have trouble with their feet throughout their entire lives.

How quickly can abnormal bone structure be changed?
The speed with which faulty bone structure can be changed to
normal depends upon the amount of vitamin D given, the adequacy of the diet in all other respects, the age of the child, the
rate of growth, and a number of other factors. In general, the
younger the child, the faster his growth, the more completely
adequate his diet, the more quickly his skeletal development
will become normal.

A year ago I saw twin girls 6 months old whose bone structure
was quite faulty. The mother had been afraid to give them cod-
liver-oil concentrate regularly because they sometimes choked
on it; when she gave it, they often threw it up. One baby's face
was narrow across the eyes, and her forehead was high and
elongated, an abnormality so obvious that the parents called her
little bunny face. The facial bones of the other baby had failed
to develop outward, giving her a shallow look which caused the
parents to be afraid she was not going to be intelligent. The
babies' ribs, chests, and legs, however, were almost normal. The
mother immediately changed to raw certified milk, increased the
amount of vitamin D, and gave it and orange juice daily without
fail. After 6 months, their facial bones were well developed, and
they are now beautiful children.

I have frequently seen the narrow, pinched faces and hollow
chests of children 2 to 5 years old become round and well formed
within 1 year after the diet has been made adequate. Between the
ages of 7 and 10, it is usually necessary for children to stay on a

complete diet for 2 years; for still older children, 3 years may be required.

It is often hard for parents to conceive of changes in facial structure sufficiently important to affect general appearance. They do not doubt, however, that their children will grow taller and their shoulders broaden. The bones of the skull, face, and jaws will broaden in the same way and proportionately to the same extent that width is gained across the shoulders.

I shall never forget a small 12-year-old boy brought to me by his mother at the close of a lecture. The child had a weaselly little face which appeared to be all eyes and crooked teeth. The mother had taken him to three orthodontists and had been given prices ranging from $1,100 to $1,500 for straightening his teeth, money which she could ill afford to spend though she felt she had to. She wanted to know if an adequate diet would allow his jawbones to develop to the extent that his teeth would straighten themselves. I answered that it was worth trying; orthodontia, if necessary, could be started when he was 15. Since the mother was well informed on nutrition and so much money was involved, his diet was kept more than adequate. Probably few children have ever drunk so much fresh orange juice and certified milk or eaten so many foods prepared with powdered milk and wheat germ; in addition he was given a capsule supplying 25,000 units of vitamin D every Sunday and Wednesday which allowed him approximately 7,000 units of the vitamin per day. I did not see the boy again for 2 years. In the meantime he had grown tremendously and was both tall and broad for his age. His facial bones were beautifully developed, his teeth were absolutely even, and he was so handsome I could scarcely believe he was the same child I had seen before. Aside from food which would have been purchased in any case, this form of "orthodontia" had cost $4 for vitamin D.

The fallacy of mechanical orthodontia is that it can improve only the jawbones. When the diet is kept adequate, however, the teeth and all the bones in the body can be improved and the general health as well.

How much vitamin D should be given? No one knows how much vitamin D is needed to promote ideal bone structure. An infant or child who grows slowly requires less than a rapidly growing one. An individual will need more of the vitamin during periods of rapid growth than when growth is slow. The more calcium obtained in the diet, the smaller the amount of vitamin D required. When the vitamin is diluted, as in an aqueous solution added to milk, it is absorbed more completely than in a concentrated form.

Most pediatricians recommend that normal infants and children be given daily 5 to 10 drops of cod-liver-oil concentrate supplying 900 to 1,800 units of vitamin D. Since you may sometimes forget to give it, or the baby may spit it up, or all of the vitamin may not be absorbed, the large number of units is probably preferable, whether given in oil or in aqueous solution.

Vitamin D is toxic if too much is given. Vomiting and diarrhea may occur; calcium becomes so easily dissolved that much of it is lost in the urine, and some may even be laid down in the soft tissues. If the toxic dose is continued, death can result. Many studies indicate that toxicity does not occur unless the vitamin is given daily to infants over an extended period in quantities of 20,000 to 40,000 units [4] and approximately ten times that amount to adults (ref. 2, p. 39).

Because of fear of toxicity, the common error has been to give too little vitamin D rather than too much. Experiments in which varying amounts of the vitamin D were given to children with tooth decay showed that the amount of decay did not decrease when less than 2,000 units of the vitamin were given daily. Dr. Johnston, pediatrician in chief at the Henry Ford Hospital in Detroit (ref. 1, p. 210), in working with older children found that when vitamin D was increased from 2,000 to almost 4,000 units daily, larger amounts of calcium were retained with the larger doses of the vitamin. Much more research is needed before the ideal amount of vitamin D will be known.

[4] S. G. Ross and W. E. Williams, "Vitamin D Intoxication in Infancy," *Am. J. Dis. Child.*, 58 (1939), 1142.

A number of studies [5] have been made in which infants were given single doses of 300,000 units or more of vitamin D by mouth; in no case have such single doses been toxic. They have, however, been found to prevent rickets for 6 months or longer. Such studies indicate that the vitamin is stored if large enough quantities are obtained and suggest an easy way for the vitamin to be given.

Vitamin-D preparations which also contain vitamin A are undoubtedly best for infants and small children. When youngsters get older, the cheapest and easiest way I know of to give the vitamin D is in capsules of 25,000 units each. One of these capsules each week appears to be sufficient for any children under 7 or for an older child whose bone and dental development is normal. For older children whose bones are underdeveloped or whose teeth are crowded together, I have recommended one of these capsules after breakfast every Wednesday and Sunday and vitamin A, when needed, in separate capsules. Over a period of 10 years or more I have watched dozens of underdeveloped children who are taking this quantity of vitamin D; I have never known of one who did not become immeasurably more attractive and whose teeth did not straighten without orthodontia as long as other bone-building nutrients were also supplied.

Let us stop depending on sunshine as a source of vitamin D. Let us give our children a chance to be beautiful by seeing that their diets supply adequate amounts of all nutrients needed to build bones. Let us particularly remember that no economy is so false as an attempt to save money by not buying adequate vitamin D; that no economy is so sound as buying a dependable preparation of this vitamin for our children both summer and winter throughout their entire growth period. Few foods offer so much for so little.

[5] D. Krestin, "The Prophylaxis of Rickets by Single Massive Doses of Vitamin D," *Brit. Med. J.*, 1 (1945), 78.

CHAPTER 20

TRY TO PREVENT ALLERGIES

THERE are two things to remember about allergies: first, that
the diagnosis may be incorrect; second, that when the diet is
made adequate, an allergy frequently disappears. A children's
allergist recently told me that many mother-diagnosed allergies
were actually chronic infections which readily cleared up under
proper medical treatment. I myself have seen dozens of cases of
"allergic" eczema disappear as soon as the diet is made adequate
in all the B vitamins. It is now recognized that the common
"allergy" to egg white is often nothing more than a deficiency of
the B vitamin, biotin. Whenever an allergy is suspected, therefore,
go to your physician for an accurate diagnosis. Regardless of
what the diagnosis may be, see that the diet is adequate in every
respect.

Several months ago I saw a 13-year-old girl who had suffered
from allergies since birth. Her mother brought a list of 65 substances, mostly foods, pollens, and dandruffs, to which the child
was allergic. The parents had spent thousands of dollars in medical bills trying to help her. Twice the father had given up good
positions and had taken his family into different communities,
hoping to escape pollens which affected the girl. The mother
avoided two dozen or more foods in her cooking; yet the allergic
symptoms persisted. The child had never been allowed to eat like
other children. Food at birthday parties or meals at restaurants or
friends' homes was not for her. Yet after her diet had been made
completely adequate, her allergic symptoms gradually disappeared and have not recurred. Such a case is not unusual. If
steps could have been taken to prevent her allergies or to correct

them when they first appeared, perhaps the years of suffering, expense and worry could have been avoided.

There are many causes of allergies: psychological, environmental, and dietary, or a combination of all three. The allergy itself may appear in any number of forms of which asthma, hives, hay fever, eczema, and allergic bronchitis and rhinitis (stuffy or drippy nose) are only a few. All allergies, however, have one thing in common: an irritant, spoken of as an antigen, gets into the blood and causes specific symptoms to occur. The offending substance may be house dust, dandruff from almost any animal, pollens from plants, or bits of incompletely digested foods. Why these substances should affect one person and not another or why they affect a person differently at different times, no one knows.

Keep vitamin C more than adequate. In numerous experiments, allergies have been induced in animals by injections of foreign materials; when vitamin C has been given before the offending substance, allergic reactions have been prevented; other animals given identical injections but no vitamin C suffer severe allergic reactions or die of anaphylactic shock. Before the injections are given, the amount of vitamin C, however, must be many times that normally needed. The blood of persons suffering from allergies has also been found to be extremely low in this vitamin even when large amounts are taken. Vitamin C appears to act as a detoxifying agent against any foreign substance which gets into the blood.[1] If this vitamin is generously supplied at the time when an antigen, or material capable of causing an allergy, has access to the body, the offending substance can apparently be rendered harmless.

Persons suffering from allergies have been given varying quantities of vitamin C, ranging from 200 or 300 milligrams daily (usually too little to be of value) up to 1,500 milligrams daily (maybe more than is needed). Since the amount of vitamin C desirable appears to be in proportion to the quantity of antigen which has gained access to the blood, the amount of the vitamin

[1] H. R. Rosenberg, *Chemistry and Physiology of Vitamins* (rev. reprint; New York: Interscience Publishers, Inc., 1945), p. 330.

needed cannot be known but varies with each person and each allergic attack. The only safe procedure appears to be to err on the side of giving more vitamin C than needed rather than too little.

It is probably wise to give an infant or child who is subject to allergies no less than 300 milligrams of vitamin C daily. This amount can be added to a baby's formula or given to an older child in fruit juice. During an acute allergic attack, large amounts of vitamin C (as much as 1,000 milligrams, or 10 tablets of 100 milligrams each) have been given to infants and children at the onset, followed every 2 hours by 200 or 300 milligrams of the vitamin. In such cases, the tablets should be melted in boiling water (p. 132), sweetened to taste, and given in juice.

The benefits of giving large amounts of vitamin C vary widely but are at times spectacular. I recently saw a 3-year-old girl suffering so severely from hay fever that she literally rained tears. I immediately gave her 1,000 milligrams of vitamin C in ¼ cup of pineapple juice. In a few minutes her tears diminished and within ½ hour she showed no signs of allergy. Other children, however, may be apparently unaffected by the vitamin.

The extent to which the need for vitamin C varies is shown by the following case history. Some time ago I saw a 4-year-old boy who had suffered from allergies since birth. Although he was allergic to many pollens and foods, his most serious allergy was to horse dandruff. Ironically his parents were show-horse people. Most of his symptoms disappeared within a few weeks after his diet was improved. He gained weight and seemed quite normal except on every fourth week end when it was necessary for his parents to take him to certain stables. On these occasions, his symptoms returned, he suffered nose bleeds, and his mother reported that he would be literally covered with bruises during the next few days. Even though he was already getting 100 milligrams of vitamin C with each meal, the bruises and nose bleeds indicated that this amount of the vitamin was not enough to protect him when exposed to a large amount of horse dandruff. I suggested that the mother give him 100 milligrams of vitamin C almost every hour, starting the day they planned to take him into the danger zone and continuing until he was home again. Since this procedure has been followed, no allergic symptoms have recurred during a number of trips to the stables.

Whenever an offending substance, or antigen, is known, this same procedure might be followed by any mother. For example, if a child is allergic to egg white, it might be wise to give him extra vitamin C before he goes to a birthday party where cake containing egg white will probably be served. When a child is affected by pollens, extra vitamin C might be given before taking him for a ride in the country. In case a youngster is allergic to cat or dog hair, he may profit by taking vitamin C before going to play with a friend who has a kitten or a puppy. Since bleeding and inflamed gums indicate a lack of vitamin C, watch for these symptoms and increase the child's intake of this vitamin whenever either condition becomes evident.

Possible relation of other nutrients to allergies. Almost every nutrient has been reported as helping allergies in humans or preventing induced allergies in experimental animals. This list includes diets high in fat, protein, calcium, and other minerals, vitamins A, C, D, E, P, and the B vitamins. The only consistency about such reports is that they have been inconsistent: one person may be helped by the particular nutrient, whereas another with similar allergic symptoms may not be. Probably the person who benefited was deficient in that nutrient, and the one unaffected was already adequately supplied with it.

Large amounts of vitamin A have been helpful in treating certain cases of hay fever, allergic rhinitis and bronchitis, and certain food allergies. In the treatment of hay fever, as much vitamin A as 50,000 units has been given after each meal. The results have been good especially when the large amounts of vitamin were started 1 or 2 months before the hay-fever season sets in. Vitamin D and calcium have been used in treating both asthma and hives. More recently vitamin B₁₂ is reported as helping persons suffering from asthma. Dr. Emmett Holt, Jr. (ref. 2, p. 113) states that allergic babies are often helped more by taking sugar out of their formulas and increasing the fat than by avoiding a suspected antigen. He also brings out that anaphylactic shock and asthmatic attacks in animals can be reduced by restricting liquids or made worse by giving too many liquids.

Allergies are probably less understood than almost any other abnormality. If one can be permitted, however, to speculate from the known to the unknown, a pastime spoken of as "arm-chair science," the possible relation of nutrition to allergies becomes clearer. For example, it is known that vitamin A is necessary to maintain the health of the mucous membranes lining all the body c . es; this vitamin appears to be helpful principally in treating es which affect these membranes. When the vitamin is so rously supplied that mucous membranes are healthy, antigens have no effect on them. Healthy mucous membranes in the l passages may also prevent antigens such as pollens, dust, d dandruff from getting into the blood, and similarly healthy membranes in the digestive tract may help to keep incompletely digested food from passing through the intestinal wall to cause allergy.

It is now known that allergies are psychosomatic diseases which most readily occur when persons are emotionally upset. One reason artificially fed babies more often suffer from allergies than do breast-fed infants may be the fact that while they are being fed, they are less often held, rocked, cuddled, sung to, and made to feel secure. Experiments have shown that persons deficient in any one of a number of B vitamins worry easily, become depressed, and are readily upset emotionally. A child undersupplied with the B vitamins, therefore, may be susceptible to allergies, whereas he might be able to endure psychological upsets if he were better nourished. Furthermore, food allergies are usually caused by bits of incompletely digested food getting into the blood. When the B vitamins are undersupplied, less hydrochloric acid is produced in the stomach, smaller quantities of other digestive juices are secreted, fewer digestive enzymes are produced, and the movements necessary to mix the food with digestive juices and enzymes decrease in number. Thus a lack of these vitamins allows more food to remain undigested than when the diet is adequate. The bits of undigested food which cause allergies might have been completely digested if the B vitamins had been generously supplied.

It is known that when vitamin C is inadequate, capillaries break; that if vitamin P is undersupplied, the walls of blood vessels become porous. Perhaps antigens gain access to the blood through openings in broken capillaries caused by vitamin-C deficiency or the holes formed when too little vitamin P is obtained. Too much liquid may make allergies worse by washing vitamins C and P and the B vitamins out of the body. Since calcium, if well absorbed by the aid of abundant vitamin D, helps to relax nerve and muscle tissue, this vitamin and mineral have been given in the hope of minimizing the spasms which occur in the tiny air passages in asthma.

It is known that the tissues of persons suffering from allergies are usually water-logged; that when protein is undersupplied, waste-laden fluids cannot be withdrawn from the body; and that persons are often allergic to so many foods rich in proteins that their diets may be almost completely lacking in this essential nutrient. It is also known that if protein is inadequate, vitamin C has no effect in detoxifying an antigen. Furthermore, in experimentally induced allergies, antibodies made of protein help to protect animals from offending antigens. Antibodies may play an important role in preventing allergic reactions in humans, yet antibodies cannot be produced unless the protein in the diet is adequate. It is probably correct to say that no allergic condition can be permanently improved unless the protein in the diet is generously supplied.

We might thus go through all the known nutrients and speculate on their possible relation to susceptibility to allergies. In all probability, every nutrient necessary for health is needed to build protection against these abnormalities.

See that the diet is adequate in every respect. Until more is understood about these abnormalities, it seems to me there is only one rule to follow: see that the diet of any child suffering from allergies is more than adequate in every known nutrient. As nearly as possible, use only natural, unrefined foods in order that nutrients still unknown may also be supplied. Any nutrient which may help the particular allergy, such as vitamin A in a case of rhinitis or calcium in case of asthma, should be given in especially generous amounts, as should any other nutrient the child appears to have been deficient in. A nutrient which may be the least expected to help may be of the greatest value.

About 2 years ago a mother brought her 6-year-old daughter to see me. Since babyhood the child had suffered almost every type of allergy and had spent more time in hospitals than out, more days at home than at school. She went to school, however, whenever her wheezing was not severe in the morning. The family had moved near the ocean to escape pollens, but when the afternoon fog came in, the child's asthma became so severe that she had to be kept in a room with all windows closed. If the girl played with other children or became excited enough to run, she went into a coma and had to be given adrenalin. The mothers and even the older children in the neighborhood had been trained to say, if they saw her running, "Helen, walk. Walk." I have never seen a child who had learned to remain so completely motionless.

After the mother took a series of my lectures on nutrition, she improved the child's diet to include generous amounts of protein, fat, calcium and most of the vitamins. The allergic symptoms did not change. Since the child's principal difficulty appeared to be a lack of oxygen, and vitamin E has been found to decrease the body's need for oxygen, I suggested that capsules supplying 60 milligrams of vitamin E, or alpha tocopherol, be given her after each meal. The girl did not miss another day of the remaining 4 months of school, and only slight allergic symptoms have occasionally recurred.

Another mother, who had taken the same series of lectures and knew of Helen's case, had a small son with allergic eczema which an improved diet so far had not affected. This mother asked me if I thought vitamin E would help her son; although I told her that I doubted it, she gave the vitamin anyway. The eczema, which the child had had for almost 3 years, cleared up immediately and has not returned. In both cases, the generally improved diets probably did much to prevent the return of severe allergic symptoms. I have seen many cases of asthma which appeared to be particularly helped by vitamin E and other cases which were not.

When the diet is completely adequate in all respects, improvement usually follows, although it may be gradual and the reason remain unknown. If the diet becomes inadequate again at any time, however, you can expect the allergy to recur.

The fallacy of elimination diets. In certain cases of food allergies, the reaction is so severe when an offending food is eaten that it must be temporarily eliminated from the diet. On the other hand, when a child is allergic to many foods, some of them unknown, the symptoms often remain the same when several foods are denied him as when they are permitted. If he happens to be allergic to chocolate candy or some other nonessential, all well and good. If he is allergic to wheat, milk, and orange juice, however, and if adequate substitutes are not given him, his diet may become deficient in protein, calcium, vitamins C and P, and the B vitamins. His general health will probably suffer, and his allergies become worse. In time, if a deficient diet is continued, he may become tense and high-strung, suffer from infections because his resistance has been lowered, and develop faulty bone structure. In such cases, the cure soon becomes worse than the disease. It is not unusual to find children suffering from borderline scurvy or infants with actual scurvy because foods rich in vitamin C have been denied them.

It is important to realize that persons do not necessarily remain allergic to the same foods over long periods. I once heard an allergy specialist tell of a boy who always seemed to be allergic to four foods but each week tests showed that the four foods differed. Mothers not realizing this possibility sometimes have their children avoid nutritious foods for 3 years or more after certain tests have been taken.

If a diet cannot be made adequate without including foods to which a child is allergic, these foods should be given him unless the allergic reaction is markedly intensified. In most cases, this procedure is not necessary since adequate substitutes can be found; at times they cannot. A case which has always amused me was that of a German boy I saw in the spring of 1941. Although born in America, he had lived in Germany and admired Hitler. He suffered from allergic eczema and rhinitis, and his asthma was so severe that he had to sleep in a chair. Tests showed that he was allergic to almost every food. His diet consisted of rice, apple-sauce, asparagus, raisins, and tea, and his history understandably revealed every possible sign of malnutrition. An adequate diet could not be planned for him without including foods he was allergic to. Instead of becoming worse on such a diet, however, he gradually improved. A few months later, he was called in the first draft, and probably no boy ever went into the army less willingly. Although he was extremely upset, he ate large quantities of all the foods to which he had been allergic, but no allergy symptoms appeared. The army took him. This case also helped to convince me that when the diet is adequate, emotional strains can be withstood.

When nutritious foods must be eliminated. In all probability, only the child who is physically below par or who is suffering from malnutrition becomes susceptible to allergies. For this reason it is extremely important that adequate substitutes be found for any nutritious food which must be withheld from his diet. If the diet is allowed to be inadequate at any time, you can expect him to become allergic to more and more substances and his allergic reactions to increase in severity.

If a baby or child is allergic to fish-liver oil, substitute some preparation of vitamin A and D in aqueous solution. I have never known a child to be allergic to one of these preparations, but if such proves to be the case, try another brand in which a different solvent has been used. If trouble still persists, use a concentrate of carotene, which changes into vitamin A in the body, and pure viosterol, a form of vitamin D made by irradiating vegetable oils.

In case your baby is allergic to yeast, a condition which is rare indeed, ask your pediatrician or druggist about concentrates of liver or rice polishings to supply the B vitamins. Or pour water over wheat germ, let it stand overnight, use it in making the formula, or give it as drinking water. If an older child is allergic to wheat, then yeast and/or concentrates of liver or rice polishings can be given him. Avoid using the preparations containing the five cheaper B vitamins; the allergy may be helped by some of the B vitamins which such products do not supply.

When infants or children are allergic to orange juice, give grapefruit juice; or try lemon juice added to apple or pineapple juice. Since such sources will not supply sufficient vitamin C for an allergic child, tablets of the vitamin should be used in addition to the juice. Occasionally vitamin-C tablets also cause trouble. In such a case, buy another brand of tablets because the fillers which hold the tablets together are usually the offending substances, and various fillers are used by different companies.

Animals deficient in vitamin P and injected with an antigen suffer severe allergic shock, whereas they are protected from shock when the vitamin is adequate. This vitamin, therefore, may be important for your child. There is also evidence that more vitamin P is needed when generous amounts of vitamin C are given. In case of an allergy to orange juice, some vitamin P can be obtained from grapefruit, lemon, and prune juices. A concentrate of vitamin P can be prepared by discarding the outside of lemon rind, chopping the white part, boiling it in ½ cup of water per rind, and letting it stand overnight so that the vitamin can pass into the water. One tablespoon or more of this preparation can be added to an infant's formula or given him in fruit juice. If the child is allergic to lemon, ask your pediatrician about giving him some commercial concentrate of vitamin P such as rutin or hesperidin.

A bottle-fed infant, who may later be allergic to wheat, might conceivably be allergic to wheat-germ oil. In such a case, the contents of a capsule of vitamin E, or alpha tocopherol, can be squeezed directly on his tongue once each week. Vitamin E is stored so efficiently that laboratory animals are sometimes given a large amount of the vitamin only once each year. An older child can be given a vitamin-E capsule once or twice each week, perhaps after breakfast every Wednesday and Sunday.

From the standpoint of keeping the diet adequate, an allergy to milk is the most serious. Milk is not "mucus-forming" and should never be avoided unless an allergy to this valuable food is proved beyond question. Even then, a baby or child who is allergic to milk in one form can often tolerate it in another form. For example, infants are rarely allergic to the same milk after it has been made into yogurt (p. 196); during the culturing process, milk protein is partially digested by beneficial bacteria, and the offending substance may be broken down. A child may be allergic to one brand of evaporated or powdered milk and yet can tolerate another brand which was produced in a different part of the country, presumably because the cows may not have been exposed to certain offending pollens. An infant who is allergic to evaporated milk often is not allergic to raw certified milk. Various forms of cows' milk, especially yogurt and certified milk, should be tried before other substitutes are used.

Goats' milk, fresh or evaporated, is often recommended, but it is higher in sugar and lower in protein than cows' milk and hence is somewhat less desirable. Soybean milk is satisfactory as to protein content, but extra calcium should be added to it. During recent years, pediatricians have used digested proteins, or protein hydrolysates, for feeding allergic infants. Such products may prevent allergic reactions, but will not support the growth of experimental animals. When used for baby feeding, other foods rich in protein such as yeast, soybean or wheat-germ flour, or dried powdered liver should be added to the formula. Canned meats for babies have been given to infants only 2 weeks old; their use is justified when an allergy warrants it. They should be diluted and given from a bottle.

When an older child is allergic to milk, many other proteins can be substituted but rarely are in adequate amounts. In case you must deal with this problem, study the tables of food analysis (p. 278) and learn protein grams backward and forward. Proteins may be particularly important in overcoming allergies; therefore give too much protein rather than too little. In case milk, which is the only dependable source of calcium and vitamin B_2 in the American diet, must be avoided, some calcium salt, such as dicalcium phosphate, should be added to fruit juice or taken in tablets. Foods rich in vitamin B_2, such as liver, should be emphasized.

Although an allergy to eggs may interfere with a mother's cooking, it is not especially important as far as nutrition is concerned. Two tablespoons of wheat germ, for example, supplies the same amount of protein as an egg and furnishes more iron, vitamin E, and the B vitamins. Allergists have found, however, that children allergic to commercial eggs can eat fertile eggs without difficulty.

Substitutes can be found for almost any offending food. The important thing is to look for such substitutes and to see that your child is nourished far more adequately than a healthy child may need to be.

When allergies are severe. Since allergies are often caused by emotional disturbances, a psychiatrist or consulting psychologist may be more helpful than a physician. Sometimes, however, allergies are so severe that physicians, psychologists, and parents alike are desperate to know what to do next. Seemingly everything has been tried; nothing has helped. Instead of moving from one community to another in search of pollen-free breezes, as such families often do, I would advise moving to an acre of land, building up the soil, and raising your own food.

I recently talked to Mr. S. H. Barton, who formerly had a school for young children in our community. He grew fruits and vegetables for them in soil he had improved until it was rich in humus. His wife baked bread for the children, using wheat he had also grown and which was ground just before being used. The children were allowed only raw certified milk. No refined sugar or white flour was used. Fruits were served for desserts. Mr. Barton told me that most of their little students had suffered severely from allergies when they first enrolled. After a few weeks, the allergies magically disappeared.

Such reports are heard more and more frequently. I know of a number of families who have taken their allergic children to the country, bought a cow or goat, composted the soil, and produced their own food. The allergies have disappeared. Although no one knows why, parents care little about the reasons as long as their children are healthy.

If your child is potentially allergic. It is probably true that every child is potentially allergic if his diet is allowed to become deficient or if he must endure certain environmental and psychological bruises. Infants sometimes suffer from allergies during their first 24 hours, a condition said to be caused by difficult births. In all probability deficiencies in the mother's diet during pregnancy allowed the infant to become susceptible to allergies. Frequently infants 2 or 3 weeks old suffer from allergies.

A child is known to be potentially allergic whenever one or both parents or other close relative have suffered from allergies. Several physicians of my acquaintance speak of such cases as second- and third-generation malnutrition. If you have a history of allergies in your family, realize that your baby may be handicapped; keep him on the best diet possible and give him the best mothering you can in order to fulfill his psychological needs. Be particularly careful to avoid upsetting him by starting foods or potty training too early, taking his bottle away against his will, or forcing him to eat foods he does not desire. It is especially important for you to keep yourself healthy because calmness and patience are needed to prevent upsetting such a child.

Check and double check his diet and make sure that each body requirement is adequate. Err if necessary on the side of giving too much vitamin C rather than too little. Be absolutely sure that vitamin P is supplied at all times. Regardless of how bright the sunshine, give some form of vitamin D both summer and winter. Keep his diet high in protein and fat. Avoid all products containing refined sugar and white flour if you possibly can, and allow him to eat only foods known to build health. If the allergy suffered by a parent or other relative is hay fever or allergic bronchitis or rhinitis, it is probably wise to give him more vitamin A than you might do otherwise.

If the diet is kept completely adequate at all times, the chances are that allergies will never occur. If a diet is improved immediately after an allergy first manifests itself, the chances are that the allergy will soon disappear.

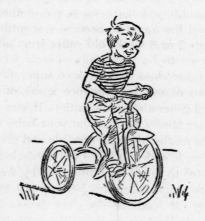

CHAPTER 21

EATING PROBLEMS
OF THE PRESCHOOL CHILD

EVERY experienced mother would probably agree that feeding an infant is a breeze compared with feeding an older child. The successful mother must be a combination of expert dietitian and psychologist and often even a detective if nutritious foods are to be eaten and appetite-destroying foods are to be kept from her child.

By the time a youngster is 2 or 3 years old, problems connected with eating often cause such a bitter clash of wills between him and his mother that he may refuse many nutritious foods merely to express his resentment. If a new baby has arrived, the mother is probably so busy and exhausted that she has little time for the older youngster and little patience with him. Certainly she may have no energy to fight with grandparents or neighbors over their filling the child up with cookies or candy. Since she no longer takes him regularly to a pediatrician, she has no one to prod her as to the adequacy of his diet. So many problems thus arise at this period that it is often spoken of medically as the neglected age.

Let us see if we can find means by which such problems may be prevented.

Improve your own food habits. Every mother knows only too well the influence her husband's food habits have upon those of her children. Hundreds of times one hears the remarks: "Their father will eat only white bread. So the children won't touch whole-wheat," or "My husband hates vegetables, hence the children refuse them too. What can you do?"

Faulty food habits on the part of the father undeniably create

real problems. Few mothers, however, have the slightest aware-
ness of the influence their own food habits have upon those of
their children. A child is with his mother more than with his
father and her influence on the child is greater than his. What is
more, she can improve her food habits if she will; her husband's,
she perhaps cannot change.

When a mother brings a child to me with the complaint that he
will not drink milk or take yeast or eat liver or any other nutritious
food, I ask her, "How much milk do you drink? Do you take
yeast? How often do you eat liver?" After a moment to recover
from surprise, most mothers admit that they avoid milk perhaps
for fear of putting on weight or that they dislike liver or yeast. I
invariably advise such mothers to make many more changes in
their own diets than in the diets of their children. Totally aside
from the child's needs, you should have an adequate diet for your
own sake. Only a healthy mother can have the energy and understanding which are demanded of her during the years her children
are growing up.

Youngsters want to grow up to be like their parents. Furthermore, they are naturally imitative. When they see you eat a food
day after day, they usually take the eating of that food for granted
and fall into line without any difficulty. On the other hand, if
you try to force a food on them which they have never seen you
eat, you can expect resistance. The mother's own food habits are
so important that they can be the factor in determining whether
her child will remain in abundant health or suffer from years of
illnesses. The place to start in either preventing or correcting poor
eating habits, therefore, is with yourself. Eat all the foods you
expect your child to eat, not just occasionally, but day after day.

Temporary dislikes for food. If the baby between 1 and 2
years old has been so fortunate as to have no unpleasant associations with food, he will probably eat like a glutton, and few or
no feeding problems arise. There may be periods when he seems
to have an off-again-on-again philosophy. He may want cottage
cheese, for example, for breakfast, lunch, and dinner one week
and refuse to touch it the next week, but before long he is eating

it again. The sooner the child can be fed from the family table, the less disconcerting these periods of refusing a formerly favorite food will be to the mother. Avoid urging him to eat some food he does not want. Instead, substitute a similar food for the disliked one, or if the food is particularly important for his health, let it go until another time and see that he becomes hungry enough to enjoy it again.

Soon after the child is 2 years old, there comes a period of negativism when he wishes to run his own life to an amazing extent. During this period he may scream No when you offer any number of formerly favorite foods; ask him if he wants a million dollars, and he will scream No with equal vigor. His refusal to eat certain foods actually has little or no relation to the foods themselves; it is merely his means of telling you he is growing up. Allow him to have only foods which can build health, but aside from this rule let him eat what and as much as he chooses. Tolerance and understanding will go farther than any amount of urging him to eat.

As the child becomes older, his rate of growth slows down, and his need for food decreases accordingly; feeding problems arise as this decrease occurs. A child of 3 years, getting all the food he needs, may eat about half as much as he ate when 18 months old. The mother, who has become accustomed to seeing him eat heartily, begins to worry when his food intake decreases even though she has been forewarned again and again that such a decrease is to be expected. The chances are that many foods which the child ate readily before he was 2 years old will be avoided at least for temporary periods between the ages of 2 and 3; that still more foods, accepted the previous year, will be frequently refused from the third to the fourth year.

If the child continued to eat as he did when he was 18 months old, he would become disgustingly fat. I recently interviewed a miserable young man who weighed over 300 pounds. He blamed his obesity on his mother, who, he said, was never happy unless she was stuffing him with food. You do not want your child to be fat when he is young or to have the problem of fighting fat when he becomes an adult. His eating patterns are being formed when he is 2 and 3 years old; let him form them, not you. A large proportion of adults who are overweight or who must continually fight fat have this problem because a clean-up-your-plate policy was strictly imposed upon them as young children, and, since early habit patterns are difficult to break, they have cleaned up their plates ever since.

As the child's food intake decreases, it is only natural that he will avoid the foods he cares the least for. In case he refuses a number of foods which you have been told repeatedly are essential to his health, you may visualize his becoming ill and will probably react by urging him to eat or perhaps even forcing him to do so. His reaction, in turn, will depend upon his personality; if he has the fortitude you want him to have, he will probably fight back tooth and nail. Such are the makings of feeding problems.

There are a number of points to remember at this stage. First, if you do not make an issue of his eating a particular food, his dislike for that food is almost always temporary. Second, avoid the statement, "Johnnie won't eat cereal" or string beans or whatever food he is currently refusing. When you make such a statement, you give the child a reputation to live up to, and it is likely that he will continue to avoid that food. Ignore his refusal or pass the matter off casually with some such remark as, "There are times when I don't feel like eating cereal either, and then at other times it tastes delicious." He may eat it the next time you serve it. It seems to me that the best attitude for a mother to take (even though it is not realistic) is to assume that every intelligent person likes all nutritious foods.

Other expressions can also be harmful. Would you eat a food you dislike, brains for example, if someone said to you, "Eat it. It's *good!*" May a curse fall upon any mother who even once utters the statement, "You must eat it. It's good for you." Children know what foods they enjoy, and at this age they care nothing about what is good for them. Such statements only arouse resentments.

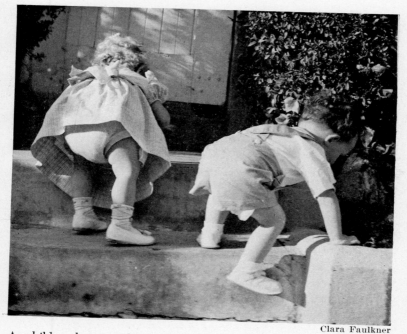

Clara Faulkner

As children become older, their rate of growth slows down and their need for food decreases accordingly. They become increasingly more interested in doing and less interested in eating.

Self-selection of foods. The famous experiment conducted by Dr. Clara M. Davis in allowing babies and small children to select their own diets is probably familiar to many of you. In this study, several babies 6 months old, who had not been given any food except milk, were allowed to eat what they preferred from a wide variety of natural foods: whole milk, both sweet or sour, and buttermilk; hard-cooked eggs; various meats, fish and fish roe; a variety of cooked cereals; fruit juices and raw and cooked vegetables and fruits. No food was salted, but salt was kept on the trays so that any child might take as much as he desired. Foods were not combined in any way; for example, grains were served only as a cereal, not as bread.

The children were fed separately and were not allowed to watch while others ate; imitation, therefore, was ruled out. Although a nurse was with each child during his meals, no attempt was made to offer him food; if a child tried to drink milk from a glass which he could not easily handle, the nurse would help but nothing more. All foods were weighed before being served, and any food left or dropped on bibs or floor was collected and weighed.

Many interesting points were brought out by this experiment. For example, one baby was allergic to egg white; this child carefully separated yolks from white, ate the yolks, and tossed the whites on the floor. All of the children went on food binges. They would sometimes drink quarts of milk one day and eat little else; the next day they would perhaps scarcely taste milk. One child ate eleven eggs at one meal; another ate thirteen bananas at one time. Again and again certain foods would be avoided for a period and then eaten heartily. The salt would sometimes not be touched for days and then eaten by the handful, even though the children grimaced as they ate it. On one day a child would perhaps eat little food of any kind; the next day he might eat tremendous quantities. Taken on the basis of day to day, the diets were lopsided indeed. When the total food consumption over a period of months was studied, however, it was found that the children ate foods supplying the nutrients they needed. No child was ill during the experiment or suffered the slightest deviation from health. Not one child had even a mild cold; none was constipated. In fact, all the children became unusually healthy.

What can we, as mothers, learn from this experiment?

First, if a food is unrefined and known to be rich in nutrients, it is probably safe to allow a child to eat as much of it as he desires without fear of allergies or digestive upsets.

Second, if a variety of foods which can build health is offered, a child will probably take good care of himself. That *if*, however, is a big one, almost an impossible one. These children were not given a grain of refined sugar on or in any food. They were not given white bread, polished rice, refined products such as cereals, macaroni, spaghetti, noodles, or crackers—even graham crackers. They were not given canned foods or warmed-over foods. Certainly they were not given jelly, jam, candy, cookies, cake, ice cream, soft drinks, pastries, desserts, and dozens of other health-destroying foods. If you have the character and the ability to duplicate the restrictions of this experiment, you can relax and be fairly sure your children will be healthy.

Third, if a child is not urged to eat and is not scolded, nagged, or prodded during his meals, he will eat heartily of his own accord. The study thus bears out what child psychologists have told us for years. During this entire experiment, not one word about a food was ever uttered while the children ate. Can you maintain such a record?

The tense, nervous child cannot take it. The husky youngster who can accept occasional prodding during meals without being upset by it usually eats heartily, and his mother, unworried, rarely bothers him. The thin, nervous child with a poor appetite is the very one who is most upset by prodding and should be allowed to eat in peace, yet it is this child who is criticized and urged to eat. The urging usually makes him tense and perhaps resentful, causing him to eat less. Such a child will want to eat between meals when the nagging has stopped and he can relax. The mother believes that he must eat something. Since wholesome food is not always available between meals, she may give him crackers or cookies. His appetite for the next meal is ruined, and he eats still less; thus the prodding is increased. A vicious circle is set up which becomes continually worse unless procedures are changed.

A similar situation often occurs after an illness. The child may have become thin and his appetite poor. Perhaps he still does not feel well, and his digestion is probably below par. His parents, impatient for his complete recovery, urge him to eat without realizing that in his condition he is most easily upset by their urging.

In my opinion there is one rule to follow on such occasions: allow your child to eat only foods which can build health, both at meals and between meals; then let him eat whatever amount he chooses. I doubt that there is anything parents must do which is more difficult than to keep quiet while an unhealthy child eats little or nothing. If they can only be patient, however, and maintain the silence of the stars, the tense child will relax or the ill one recover; soon they will have no reason to worry about his health.

Eating problems are often imagined. Not long ago I interviewed a nutrition-conscious mother who told me she was "worried sick" about her 3-year-old daughter. The child was husky and the picture of health, but she "simply wasn't eating a thing." At dinner the night before the mother had served her meat, two vegetables, salad, milk, and fruit, and the child had touched nothing except her milk. She usually ate a fair breakfast: a glass of orange juice, some cereal (or egg), and milk. She took cod-liver-oil concentrate after breakfast. During the remainder of the day she drank 1 quart of homogenized milk to which the mother had added ½ cup of powdered milk; also she took two large glasses of pineapple juice into each of which 1 heaping tablespoon of yeast had been stirred. Although the mother admitted that she should not have done so, she could not refrain from urging the child to eat. As a result their meals had become nightmares.

Obviously the mother was overdoing a good thing and expecting the child to eat far too much, though she was getting more than her requirement of 1,200 calories daily. The milk-yeast binge was probably temporary, and the diet was quite adequate as it was. I suggested that if the mother thought it necessary for the child to eat other foods, she should discontinue giving the powdered milk and should restrict the yeast-in-juice to 1 glass.

When mothers have studied nutrition perhaps with the Red Cross, I find similar problems. Such mothers often try to stuff their children with the so-called basic-seven foods. If the children refuse, the mothers are upset and start fussing with them to eat. In these cases where candy and refined foods are rarely given, the children themselves often select a more adequate diet in my opinion than do the mothers.

Let the child select the amount of food he desires. You determine what foods he can select.

Restrictions acceptably imposed. The psychologists have been trying to convince mothers that they should stop nagging, prodding, fussing, bribing, and other unpleasantness which causes the child to become tense during his meal. Criticism and scolding can upset him to the extent that his digestion is interfered with and, in all probability, allergies are often induced by this means.

Imagine that you are a child and that two giants sit beside you, criticizing you. If anyone interfered with us the way many mothers interfere with their children during meals, we could probably think only of how much we disliked that person. Certainly we would not eat heartily regardless of how hungry we might have been before we came to the table. Our children feel the same way except that their reaction may be intensified because they are young and sensitive.

On the other hand, when children are allowed to eat as they please, some of them try to get away with murder. Many will skip a meal completely to play cowboy or watch television. As soon as you have cleared the table, they want something to eat. I think most experienced mothers will agree that there must be a desirable middle road between too many restrictions and no restrictions. Let us, therefore, try to make some general rules.

A technic which seems to me to work like magic is this: every time you are tempted to criticize your child's eating, or to urge him to eat more, look for something to praise instead. For example, if you start to say, "Nancy, eat your squash," bite your tongue and say instead, "Doesn't Nancy eat nicely, Daddy? See, she has finished all her string beans." If the serving of squash has been small, chances are it will soon disappear. Praise, praise, and more praise not only helps to satisfy the child's recognition drive but lets him enjoy his meals. If you can find nothing to praise, it is worth letting a child eat little or miss a meal; then he will eat so heartily at the next meal that you can praise him.

Keep your servings small, especially when a food is unfamiliar; give the child a chance to ask for a second helping. If the food is definitely disliked, disguise it or serve no more than one to three bites until the child learns to enjoy it, even though it may be months before he does.

During the meals, try hard to treat the child as a guest. We do not urge guests to eat or to clean up their plates, and certainly we do not go into long harangues as to how a particular food will give them pearly teeth.

When restrictions necessary to cover any problem lead to bickering at mealtime, they should be discussed between meals. They should not be discussed during a meal or with any show of emotion on the part of the mother. As soon as the child is old enough to be reasoned with, make clear to him any rules or restrictions you wish to impose and the punishment or withdrawal of privilege which will follow if he does not comply with the ruling. For example, you may wish him to observe one or more of the following restrictions: to taste every food served; to remain seated throughout the meal; or to finish his meal with the members of the family. Explain that if he does not comply, he cannot stay up to watch the television tonight or play with Johnny this afternoon or what have you; that children who do not eat need more rest or cannot play as strenuously as when they have eaten. If he complies with the ruling, praise him at mealtime. Otherwise avoid the subject completely until the next midmeal period; then you might comment casually that since he did not eat some of every food served, the privilege would be withdrawn. Withdraw that privilege without fail.

When this method is used, the rule is quickly learned; the child is not made tense or antagonistic during his meal; his digestion is not interfered with. Since an interval passes between the child's failure to comply and the discussion, the mother is rarely angry or upset. Battles over particular foods, which so frequently cause a child to dislike those foods permanently, are thus avoided.

When a child dawdles over his meals too long, it is often wise to remove all food at the end of ½ hour and to give him nothing until the next meal; the procedure can be repeated if necessary. This problem, however, should first be discussed at a midmeal period, and the child warned that his food will be taken away.

The children themselves not only thrive on the praise they receive but are tremendously relieved when a policy of scolding at meals changes to one of politeness. Often an increase in appetite occurs within 2 or 3 days.

When a mother is tempted to nag, it is well to remember that most primitive people prepare a meal only once a day. Even when food is abundant, some races train their children to go without food for as long as 3 days at a time. Yet their children are far healthier than ours because the foods they eat can build health and they are not upset during meals by being nagged at.

"My child won't eat." Every health worker has heard the statement, "My child won't eat," hundreds of times. As a rule, such a statement is sheer nonsense. The mother means that the child will not eat the foods she wants him to eat or will not eat them in the amount she thinks necessary. Almost invariably such a child has been given far too many sweets and has had too many battle-royals imposed on him during meals.

Recently a mother, whom I have known for years and who could not eat intelligently if she had to, brought a gray butterball of a child to see me because "he just won't eat a thing." For breakfast she had given him orange juice, cereal, egg, toast, and milk; he had not touched any of it except to take a sip of orange juice.

In outlining such a breakfast, the mother was saying to herself, in effect, "You can see I'm doing my part. It's not my fault that he isn't healthy." Between meals the child, only 2 years old, would go to the bread drawer for bread and doughnuts which he ate in large amounts. The bread was white because the mother did not like "that brown stuff," and she purchased doughnuts because she enjoyed them for breakfast. She confessed to the usual prodding and fussing at mealtime, yet she failed to admire the child's gumption or to see that she was forcing him to take the course he did. Serving the best meals possible does not excuse this mother or any other for producing ill health in a child.

In such a case you invariably find that the child is eating something. Often the mother will say, "Yes, he drinks lots of milk," or "He'll eat as much meat as I'll let him." Perhaps he loves hot dogs and peanut butter and will tolerate peas, several fruits, and a few other really nutritious foods.

When such a problem arises, the first thing to do is not to mention food at mealtime. Allow the child to have absolutely no refined sugar or starch in any form, at meals or between meals. If he is drinking so much rich milk that he is crowding out other foods, buy milk which is not homogenized and for a few days pour off most or all of the cream. Restrict fats in other forms; add little butter to his vegetables. Serve the wholesome foods he enjoys and allow him to eat as much of them as he wants, even if it means hot dogs and peas three times a day. After a few days, have a midmeal discussion of rules and privileges. Keep his midmeals small and restrict them to food which can build health. The chances are that his appetite will quickly improve.

When the appetite is really poor. If a poor appetite continues, the child should be taken to a pediatrician and a dentist for thorough physical and dental examinations. The child may have an infection which you have not suspected. He may have worries or allergies which your physician may discover. Toxins from a dead or abscessed tooth may be draining into his blood.

Whenever the appetite is poor, your greatest emphasis must be on serving foods rich in all the B vitamins (p. 29). Serve liver two or three times each week, eating it yourself and being content if your child merely tastes it at first. Put wheat germ into every food you can. See that he has yeast daily. If necessary, give him temporarily some concentrate of natural B vitamins such as an extract of rice polishings in blackstrap molasses * or one containing liver concentrate.† A teaspoon of such a preparation before each meal usually restores the appetite in a day or two.

"He won't eat vegetables." A worried mother called me recently to say that her 3-year-old would not touch any vegetables except cooked carrots, peas, and potatoes. Her problem is not unusual.

There must be basic reasons why so many children refuse vegetables. Unless you grow your own or obtain them from a gardener whose soil is rich in humus, most of the vegetables available now are almost tasteless. Poison sprays used on the vegetables cannot be washed off, and it is possible that a child's refusal to eat vegetables is sometimes an instinctive attempt to avoid these poisons.

There is all the difference in the world between the nutrients known to be in vegetables and the amount of these nutrients absorbed from the vegetables into the child's blood. Many experiments show that the softer the texture of a food, the more complete the absorption. For example, rats made deficient in vitamin A are cured much more quickly if fed cooked apricots rather than raw ones even though some of the carotene, or vitamin A, is destroyed by cooking; yet the texture of a raw apricot is not hard compared with that of many foods. Time and again you will notice that a child will eat vegetables having a soft texture and refuse the ones with coarse or hard texture. As a child grows older, his digestion becomes more efficient, and he will probably eat and absorb more nutrients from vegetables which he formerly refused.

As I see it, vegetables have no nutrients which cannot be more

* Galen B Syrup, Galen Company, Richmond, California.

† Lederplex Vitamin B Complex Liquid, Lederle Laboratories, New York, N. Y.

easily obtained from fruits. The texture of fruits is usually softer than that of vegetables; hence the nutrients they supply are absorbed in larger quantities. Fruits are less often soaked before being cooked; if they are boiled, the water is not thrown away; they are usually better sources of vitamin C than are vegetables; and if avocados, apricots, yellow peaches, yellow melons, and other yellow or green fruits are selected, they are excellent sources of carotene, or vitamin A. They supply the same minerals as do vegetables. Furthermore, most children enjoy fruits far more.

My advice to this mother was to continue to give her child one bite of any vegetables she prepared for the family, but to serve him fruits as a substitute for vegetables. Whenever she plans to serve vegetables which the child will not eat, she makes him a fruit salad or fruit cup or gives him a fresh, stewed, or canned fruit. If a variety of vegetables is eaten by other members of the family, in time the child will also eat them. I have used this procedure with our son and have been repeatedly surprised at the number of times he has eaten large amounts of vegetables he had formerly refused for months.

In my opinion, vegetables for children, particularly salads and green leafy vegetables, are greatly overemphasized. Allow your child to eat the ones he wants, and worry not at all about those he refuses.

Missing a meal. Many mothers will miss meals themselves time and again and think little of it. If their children miss a meal, however, these same mothers will raise the roof. There will be times when your child does not want to eat. If you leave him alone and do not allow him devitalized foods before the next meal, he will probably make up his loss, and little harm will be done.

This point was forcefully brought home to me once last year. I had to lecture at a dinner meeting, an hour's drive from home. The baby sitter, whom I had had many times before, arrived extremely late. Although I had our son's dinner ready to serve, in my haste to get away I thought that she knew our routine and that I need give her no instructions. On returning home, I discovered that she had put him to bed without his dinner, having assumed that he had already eaten. I felt sick. Why had I neglected him? I had no business to be lecturing when he needed me. The next morning, however, I stopped worrying. I have rarely seen a person of any age eat such a huge breakfast; it was almost impossible to fill him up.

If a child misses many meals or does not increase his food consumption at the next meal, he should be taken to a pediatrician and the cause determined. Missing an occasional meal, however, is no reason for worry.

The breakfast problem. The problem of children going without breakfast is usually the result of a combination of causes. It rarely becomes a problem until children start going to play school. Not the least of the causes is that parents and children go to bed too late and hence get up too late to have time for a leisurely breakfast. The mother, fearing that the youngsters will be late, becomes tense and usually attempts to hurry them; the tension and perhaps scolding make it difficult for them to eat. Children have no sense of time; to try to hurry them means only to confuse them. The solution to this problem is for the family to go to bed earlier and rise in time to have a relaxed, unhurried breakfast.

Another cause of the "breakfast problem" is faulty eating habits on the part of the parents. Often the father eats earlier or later or gets breakfast in town; perhaps the mother misses breakfast or prefers to eat after the child has gone to play school. Regardless of what the father does, at least a mother can sit down and have a pleasant, leisurely meal with her children if she is willing to make the effort to do so. It is up to her to set the example.

One of the main causes of a child's not wanting breakfast is that he has been given too hearty a meal in the evening and/or too sweet a dessert; he still has plenty of sugar (glycogen) stored in his body, his blood sugar is still normal, and physiologically he does not need food at breakfast time. By the middle of the morning, however, when it may be impossible for him to eat, his blood sugar will have dropped, and his need for food can become acute.

The first step in rectifying this problem is to confine desserts to unsweetened fruits or to avoid them entirely. If this procedure does not work, the next step is to see that he eats less for dinner. One of the easiest ways to cope with the problem is to give the child such a hearty midmeal in the afternoon that his appetite for dinner will be ruined. He may be permitted such foods as cheese, peanut butter, hot dog, or liverwurst sandwich on whole-wheat or wheat-germ bread; as much milk as he wants; an orange or banana or any other fruit. Let him eat as much as he wants as long as the food offered him can build health. He may eat little at dinner, but he will be ready for a hearty breakfast.

The one main cause of feeding problems. There actually is only one real cause of feeding problems: allowing a child too many refined foods. The emotional and psychological problems arise after the child's appetite and perhaps health have been ruined by such foods.

The number of foods which cannot build health is no less than staggering, and new ones appear on the market every year. The foods made from white flour, in which some twenty or more God-given nutrients have been discarded and perhaps small amounts of three nutrients (vitamin B_1, niacin, iron) have sometimes been put back, are alone sufficient to cause feeding problems. These foods include: all the bakery products made of white flour such as cakes, pies, cookies, rolls, bread, and doughnuts; the usual variety of crackers, macaroni, spaghetti, and noodles; prepared mixes for making rolls, cakes, pie dough, gingerbread, waffles, and hot cakes; the refined cereals such as farina and cream of wheat. In addition are the usual gelatin desserts which contain much sugar and water, artificial coloring and flavoring, and a little protein of extremely poor quality; all the soft drinks and preparations children are urged to use to make drinks at home; polished rice; the almost endless list of foods containing far too much appetite-satisfying refined sugar, such as candy of all varieties, jams, jellies, and oversweet desserts. There are also many foods which could not be called refined, and yet their nutrients have been largely discarded or destroyed by heat during processing.

These include many quick-cooking cereals and most of the cold cereals except shredded wheat.

A child's stomach is relatively small; his appetite is readily satisfied. Every time you allow him as much as a bite of refined food, know that a more valuable food is being crowded out. If a child's requirements of growth are to be met and superior health is to be maintained, there is no place in any dietary for a food which cannot build health. When a mother is careless in allowing devitalized foods to be eaten, she can expect not only feeding problems but deviations from health as well.

The rule to solve feeding problems. There is one rule which, when applied daily year after year, will correct or prevent most, if not all, feeding problems: restrict the foods you serve to those which can build health. The more serious the feeding problem, the more rigidly should this rule be applied.

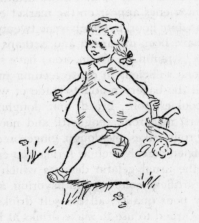

CHAPTER 22

THE CARDS ARE STACKED
AGAINST YOU

THE principal cause of the "neglected age" referred to in the previous chapter is that a child usually starts eating at the family table when he is about 18 months old. Sugar, formerly denied him, may be heaped on cereals. Devitalized foods of every kind, if prepared for the family, are allowed him. The result is that about 1 year later the abundant health he may have enjoyed as a toddler has given way to the obvious signs of malnutrition so evident in every nursery school. The truth of the matter is that the family table in the majority of American homes cannot support the health of parents or children. There is only one way you can be fairly sure of raising healthy children: to become and remain healthy parents.

Foods which build health can also be delicious. Parents often do not wish to eat the food they believe their children should eat because they consider such food unpalatable. To an intelligent person, however, a food must meet two requirements: it must taste good and must build health.

Every person will surely agree that a quickly cooked and intensely green vegetable is far more delicious than one overcooked until it resembles a rag you have used to clean the car; that a tossed salad, as crisp as snow on a frosty night, far surpasses a wilted one; that a juicy steak, so tender it can be cut with a butterknife, is superior to a tough, dry one broiled at a nutritive-destroying high temperature. Anyone who has once tasted fruits and vegetables grown in soil rich in humus will tell you that the flavor of the poor-quality products in our markets is by contrast abominable. Although you may not enjoy your first taste of yogurt, it has been eaten for centuries by gourmets the world over who probably did not give a hoot about their health.

I have heard dozens of people exclaim after tasting bread made of wheat germ and freshly stone-ground wheat, "It's as good as cake." For years I have held that no one has even tasted a decent waffle until he eats one made with whole-wheat flour, wheat germ, and bakers' yeast. Wonderful cookies and pie dough can be made of health-building ingredients. Many persons remark when eating gelatin desserts containing powdered and evaporated milk that the "whipped cream" makes these foods too rich.

Health-minded persons sometimes disapprove of the refined sugar used in such desserts. Actually, when desserts are prepared with health-building ingredients, they usually have a lower sugar content and a much higher content of protein, calcium, the B vitamins, and other nutrients than such foods as raisins and dates which these persons themselves would recommend. A craving for sweets, however, almost invariably indicates a deficiency of protein or of the B vitamins. When these nutrients are supplied, the desire for sweets diminishes or disappears. Most families whose diets are adequate serve fruits for desserts or give up desserts entirely except for special occasions mainly because they no longer care for them.

Eating foods which can build health in yourselves and your children should mean that your food will be delicious.

Fresh and inexpensive supplies are essential. It has been difficult to purchase many nutritious foods, and even when sources are located, the foods are often stale. For example, a friend who had just purchased my cookbook recently invited me to dinner. She had made yeast rolls and pie crust of wheat germ and whole-wheat flour and had used powdered skim milk in preparing a cream soup and the pie filling. These supplies, which were new to her, she had purchased at a store where calls for them were infrequent. She had not read the warning that good powdered milk has the texture of face powder and a faint odor similar to that of

fresh coconut. The milk she bought had been exposed to moisture, smelled to the high heavens, and was in marble-hard lumps.
The flour and the wheat germ appeared to have been milled about
1920 and must have been rancid and full of weevils since 1922.
Her food was embarrassingly inedible. I shudder to think of how
many persons may have had similar experiences.

Health-food stores carry powdered skim milk and wheat germ
which are fresh; they obtain whole-wheat flour from mills where
it is stone-ground daily. They also stock brewers' yeast, blackstrap molasses, and many other health-building foods. If you do
not have such a store in your community, write to the chamber
of commerce in the city nearest you and ask for the address of
such stores. Or buy wheat germ and middlings, wheat germ,
whole-wheat flour and similar products directly from one of the
excellent mills throughout the country.*

Recently many stores have stocked health-building products
but charge exorbitant prices. For example, I recently saw blackstrap molasses priced at 89 cents a quart. We buy our molasses
from a bakery supply house for 23 cents a quart by getting it in
5-gallon cans, or for $4.50 for 5 gallons instead of $17.80. My
milkman delivers powdered skim milk to me in 100-pound sacks
for $14, or 14 cents a pound and, since there is a surplus of mil-
lions of pounds of powdered skim milk in America, this wholesale
price should not increase appreciably. Most bakers use powdered
milk and blackstrap molasses, and a kindly baker will share his
supply with you at the price he pays. Although brewers' yeast is
often priced at $2 a pound or more, a market near us sells excel-
lent yeast † for 59 cents a pound.

If a price seems exorbitant to you, trace the source of supply

---

* El Molino Mills, Alhambra, California.
  The Great Valley Mills, Ivyland, Bucks County, Pennsylvania.
  Elam Mills, Chicago, Illinois.
  Wight's Grist Mill, Old Sturbridge Village, Sturbridge, Massachusetts.
  The Stone Buhr Milling Company, 3509 Evanston Street, Seattle,
    Washington.
  † Strain G, Anheuser Busch, Inc., St. Louis, Mo.

and ask the proprietor of a market to stock the food at a reasonable price; or ask a group of friends to share the food with you so that you can buy it wholesale. Most large milk companies sell powdered skim milk. If yours does not, any baker can tell you where to buy either powdered milk or blackstrap molasses. Store your powdered milk in airtight tins such as those you buy popcorn in; keep milk for your immediate use in a vacuum-pack coffee tin. I would not recommend that you buy powdered whole milk; it is too expensive and too filling. Although brewers' yeast is usually sold wholesale in lightweight drums holding 100 pounds, it keeps so well that many families buy that quantity for themselves. None of these products need to be refrigerated except perhaps wheat germ during extremely hot weather.

Fortunately such foods as brown rice and converted rice are widely available. Before converted rice * is hulled, it has been treated with steam which carried the B vitamins into the rice. If this rice is not in your market, ask your grocer to stock it. Macaroni, spaghetti, noodles, and similar products made of whole-wheat flour or whole-wheat and soy flours can usually be purchased at health-food stores only. These products are excellent when fresh. We use them so infrequently, however, that they often become stale after we have purchased them. Consequently I more often buy from the health-food stores similar products prepared for diabetic persons; these foods are made of wheat from which the starch has been removed, and only the wheat protein, or gluten, remains. Although such macaroni or noodles lack the nutrients of whole wheat, they are low in calories and high in protein, keep indefinitely and are delicious.

Rules for introducing foods. An unfamiliar flavor is rarely enjoyed. We learn to like foods only by tasting them again and again. I once heard the remark that if Americans had never tasted coffee, a coffee salesman would have one devil of a time trying to make them drink it. Many mothers become so enthusiastic about nutrition that they try to change their family's eating habits over-

* Uncle Ben's Rice, Converted Rice, Inc., Houston, Texas.

night. They usually introduce health-building foods having unfamiliar flavors in too large quantities. Sometimes they try to force their children to eat unfamiliar foods. Invariably they talk so much that they make their husbands and older children alike suspicious of everything they cook. Their methods defeat their own purpose.

Make the introduction of such foods as powdered skim milk, yogurt, wheat germ, blackstrap, and yeast *a secret game all your own.* See how far you can go in fortifying ordinary foods before anyone discovers what you are doing. Perhaps the first time you add powdered milk to fresh milk or wheat germ to a cereal, someone mentions the unusual taste. Lift a surprised eyebrow, comment casually that you are sorry and you will speak to the milkman, and that the cereal might be a bit stale, but you will hasten to buy more. Add less of the health-building food the next time. Since wheat germ and middlings cooked as a cereal supply more wheat germ with less wheat-germ flavor than almost any other food, start with it. Later, add wheat germ to cereals with which its flavor will blend most easily, such as wheat cereals rather than oatmeal.

When introducing yeast to any person who has never tasted it before, stir no more than ½ teaspoon into a large glass of juice (8 ounces). Gradually increase the amount. I have never known a child to dislike yeast when it is thus introduced gradually, especially if he is given only sips at first and praised for drinking it. When a mother has eventually increased her yeast intake to 1 tablespoon or more daily, she usually looks and feels so much better and her disposition is often so noticeably improved that her husband starts taking it. Blackstrap molasses should be similarly introduced by stirring only ¼ or ½ teaspoon into a glass of milk. An introductory serving of yogurt (p. 175) should be small and perhaps made into a sundae with honey, maple syrup, sweetened raspberries, or crushed pineapple over it.

After a flavor has become familiar, foods which are eaten most frequently are usually the ones most enjoyed. Children believe that their mothers are the best cooks in the world because they have eaten their mother's cooking most often. When health-building foods are introduced wisely and later served day after day, they soon become old favorites.

"This one time won't hurt." Any mother who tries to give her children only foods which build health will repeatedly hear the argument, "This one time won't hurt." Relatives or friends who care little about your children's health may take them on picnics or trips to the zoo or circus where they may fill up on white buns, soft drinks, or perhaps candy. On such holidays as Easter and Christmas your children may become ill because of being given sweets. There will be birthday parties where naps are interrupted and appetites are ruined. Such "one times" can multiply into dozens of times and become health hazards. The wise mother must be on her guard and be prepared for such occasions.

Nutritious lunches can be packed for picnics and trips. Children enjoy making at home holiday candies which can be far superior nutritionally to commercial varieties. There are two solutions to the birthday-party problem. One is to give the party in the morning and to serve a light lunch; the other is to give a late-afternoon party, when naps are over, and serve a light dinner or supper. A number of intelligent mothers in our community have given such parties which have been most successful. Why not set the example for your community?

There will be times, however, when you will probably want to serve refined foods. You will usually find that they do not taste nearly as good as you once thought they did. There will also be occasions when you and your children will need to eat devitalized foods to keep from insulting a hostess. There will be instances when it may harm your child's mental health more to prevent him from eating with his group than to allow him to eat foods you disapprove of. Although we hope such occasions will be infrequent, do not make yourself a bore or your child an outcast by becoming too enthusiastic about nutrition.

Foods with a bad reputation. Many foods are considered taboo for children, usually without reason. For example, Dr.

Richardson [2] searched the medical literature in vain for a scientific basis for the belief that fried foods are harmful. He then sought the opinion of pediatricians and nutritionists, but no one knew of any reason why such foods should not be given to babies. Actually most foods spoken of as fried are really sautéed, or cooked by the heat of steam, and are certainly harmless.

I once spent a day in a medical library trying to find experimental evidence indicating that herbs, spices, and other seasonings were detrimental to health. Since I found nothing, I went to several professors in a medical school and asked them. None of them knew of any way in which seasonings could be harmful. Each pointed out that herbs were probably beneficial, and two mentioned that onions and garlic were thought to contain a germicidal substance.

The argument is often used that if children are given highly seasoned foods, they no longer enjoy bland foods. The truth is that no human being could enjoy many of the bland foods offered children. Certainly a child who eats government-inspected hot dogs (a nutritious food because soy flour and powdered milk are used to hold them together) can still enjoy the subtle flavors of cream of mushroom soup and broiled lobster as much as can you or I.

Sea foods themselves are often on the taboo list, probably a hangover from the time before refrigeration was available. Most sea foods are so rich in protein, iodine, and other nutrients that it would be hard to find a better food for your baby or small child.

Many mothers are afraid to give young children the so-called gas-forming vegetables of the cabbage and onion families. These vegetables form gas only when the sulfur compounds they contain are first broken down by overcooking or by enzymes during long storage. If these vegetables are fresh and quickly cooked, there is no reason why they should not be given to a baby.

[2] F. H. Richardson, "Fried Foods for Children," *J. Pediat.*, 24 (1944), 199.

Cheeses are on an infant's forbidden list because they are supposedly constipating or "hard to digest"; actually they are neither. Processed cheeses are solidified by being hydrogenated, as are many cooking fats; hence they are lower in protein than natural cheeses. All other cheese, however, is excellent. If you are enjoying hors d'œuvres and cocktails while your toddler is reaching and begging, give him cheese instead of crackers.

Even the poor starchy foods, such as potatoes and cereals, have sometimes been slandered. As long as a food is unrefined and is prepared in such a way that the nutrients God put into it are largely retained, it usually remains an excellent food regardless of how high its starch content. One exception, however, is in using wheat germ rather than unground wheat as a cereal; since the protein, vitamins and minerals are concentrated in the germ, whereas wheat itself is about 75 per cent starch, the germ obviously has more to offer. Oatmeal has recently been threatened because it contains phytic acid which combines with calcium and prevents it from reaching the blood. If you enjoy oatmeal, cook it in milk into which powdered milk has been beaten; count some of the calcium as lost.

The only foods which should be taboo are highly refined ones or foods made of highly refined ingredients.

Balanced day or week versus balanced meals. I have never been sure what a "balanced" meal is, but it appears to be one consisting of such a large number of foods that a dab of most of the body requirements is supplied at one time. A colored fruit or vegetable furnishes a little vitamin A; whole-grain bread or cereal or meat contributes some B vitamins; a juice or fresh fruit or salad is included to prevent scurvy, and so on. To me the concept of such a meal seems wrong, nutritionally and otherwise. Large meals are expensive, tempt one to overeat, and involve too much cooking and dish washing. As long as the daily requirements are met, there is no reason why eating a small amount of several foods is preferable to eating a larger quantity of one or two health-building foods which you thoroughly enjoy.

For example, to escape evening traffic I recently dropped in for a visit with friends and shared a delicious dinner with them. Each of us had a glass or more of raw certified milk and several slices of hot home-baked bread made of wheat germ and stone-ground, whole-wheat flour. We did not speak of the meal as dinner at the time, but we later discovered that none of us had cared to eat more that evening.

Variety can be gained in a day or week rather than at a meal. When three or four vegetables are served each day, the same vegetables appear monotonously on the menus several times a week; if only one or two vegetables are served, menus can achieve interest. There is nothing wrong with one-dish meals such as a large bowl of piping-hot cereal for breakfast or a cream soup for lunch or yogurt and berries for supper provided the total daily food intake supplies your needs. Children often prefer such meals. Serve large meals if you want to, but do not feel that you must or that your family must eat them even if you wish to serve them.

Far more important than "balanced" meals is the balance of meals during the day. Breakfast need not be large but should supply 20 grams or more of protein (p. 108). The midday meal should be heavy, moderate, or light depending upon the amount of physical work to be done during the afternoon. The evening meal should be filling but light so that appetites can be ready for a breakfast. Everyone, particularly women and children, should eat midmeals to replenish the blood sugar and thus prevent a lag in energy production.

The daily plan. In case these many instructions seem more confusing than the mere business of eating has any right to be, let us see what a 1-year-old may be served during a day and how his food changes as he grows older. By this time he should have given up most canned or blended foods and be accustomed to small pieces of meat, hard-cooked egg, and cheese; to mashed, chopped, shredded, and quickly cooked vegetables; and to other foods of "adult" textures. In short, if the family table can support health, he should be eating with his parents.

ON WAKING:

milk from breast or bottle

10 drops of cod-liver-oil concentrate unless aqueous solution of vitamins is added to formula

halibut-liver oil and wheat-germ oil if used

BREAKFAST:

juice or fruit

wheat germ and middlings as a cereal (cooked in milk) or wheat germ added to any whole-grain cereal (without sugar) or stirred into fruit or served in waffles or hot cakes

egg instead of or in addition to cereal if enjoyed

toasted whole-grain or wheat-germ bread

BEFORE MORNING NAP:

milk from breast or bottle

MIDDAY MEAL:

wheat germ if none for breakfast, as a cereal or in fruit; or

meat, fish, fowl, sea food, eggs, cheese, or cream soup

1 cooked vegetable if enjoyed, or 2 if flavor of one is unfamiliar

bits of raw vegetable, as tomato, avocado, or grated vegetable if mother desires; increase variety as the child grows older

fruit or dessert made of milk (may be omitted)

BEFORE AFTERNOON NAP:

milk from breast or bottle

AFTER NAP:

citrus juice if none for breakfast

EVENING MEAL:

any combination of foods suggested for the noon meal; should include protein and a fruit or vegetable

BEFORE GOING TO SLEEP:

milk from breast or bottle

The foregoing plan purposely violates the simple-meal theory in order to include several suggestions for mothers who wonder what they can feed their children.

A baby's quota of breakfast protein would be supplied largely by the milk in the morning bottles. As a child grows older, the protein should be incorporated into breakfast itself. The easiest and cheapest method is to beat powdered milk with the fresh milk to be drunk and used on cereal. In preparing any hot cereal for the family, first stir thoroughly ½ cup of powdered milk with 1 cup of cereal, then add salt and 2 cups of liquid; put over the direct heat for a few minutes and finish cooking in a double boiler. Instead of the usual bacon and eggs, you might serve ground meat patties, hot dogs, sautéed liver, or melted cheese on toast.

When a child gives up his bottle, which we hope will not be until he is at least 3 years old, midmeals will need to be planned for him. They can still consist of milk and citrus juice as before or can be any fruit or juice, or a piece of cheese, a hot dog, or a sandwich with milk.

A child of 3 or 4 is often so active that it seems impossible to keep an ounce of fat on him. In case he has become accustomed to a cod-liver-oil concentrate and enjoys the flavor, it may be wise to supply extra calories by changing to plain cod-liver oil and gradually increasing the amount to 1 to 3 tablespoons daily, taken after a meal or after each meal. Actually old-fashioned cod-liver oil is probably superior to any of the newer concentrates. The child may, however, insist on changing to vitamin capsules if he sees his parents taking them. If this is the case, give him capsules containing both vitamins A and D or a capsule supplying vitamin A daily and one furnishing vitamin D every Sunday (p. 228), but avoid the multiple-vitamin capsules. If he turns against all forms of cod-liver oil, hide a few drops of an aqueous solution of vitamins A and D in his food.

Wheat-germ oil, in case you have been giving it, can be stopped as soon as the child is eating 1 tablespoon of wheat germ daily. If he avoids wheat germ for some time, however, better give the oil again or occasionally give him a capsule supplying vitamin E, perhaps one every 2 weeks. Yeast mixed in fruit juice or tigers' milk should be introduced from a cup or glass long before the bottle is given up. If it has not been introduced, try it now but use the patience-of-a-saint method. Give the child vitamin-C tablets or melt them and add them to juice, fruit, or milk whenever he neglects citrus juice.

Aside from these simple changes, his meal plans can stay roughly the same throughout childhood.

How much of each nutrient? Mothers invariably ask how much wheat germ, yeast, or other nutritious foods a child should eat daily. It is dangerous to answer such questions. Too many mothers try to force a child to eat a specified amount of food; resentments and feeding problems arise, and poorer health results.

Let us answer these questions by studying the daily dietary allowances recommended by the Food and Nutrition Board of the National Research Council. If you calculate the nutrients your child obtains in 1 day by using the tables of food analysis (pp.

Age of Child	Calories	Protein grams	Calcium grams	Iron mg.	Vitamin A units
Under 1 year	50 per lb.	1.6 per lb.	1	6	1,500
1 to 3 years	1,200	40	1	7	2,000
4 to 6 years	1,600	50	1	8	2,500

	Vitamin B$_1$ mg.	Vitamin B$_2$ mg.	Niacin mg.	Vitamin C mg.	Vitamin D units
Under 1 year	0.4	0.6	4	30	400
1 to 3 years	0.6	0.9	6	35	400
4 to 6 years	0.8	1.2	8	50	400

278-293) you can readily see whether his diet meets these allowances. Any mother who thinks that her child eats too little should certainly count his calories. Except for calories, iron and calcium, these allowances are low. I want my children to have about half again as much protein and about five times the suggested quantities of vitamins. I would not worry about the children if their food intake for a day met only these allowances. I would, however, prepare appetizing foods which contain the inadequate nutrients and use undercover methods to see that the children were hungrier and thirstier.

The cards are stacked against you. Despite the fact that most mothers are conscientious, and that more and more of them are applying nutrition, few children in our entire country enjoy optimum health. Tooth decay is the rule rather than the exception. Faulty posture is almost as prevalent. The incidence of infantile paralysis doubled in a single year. Heart disease and cancer, once thought of as diseases of the aged, annually take the lives of thousands of children. Multiple sclerosis, rarely heard of before Lou Gehrig died of the disease, is said to be increasing rapidly. There are many causes of these depressing conditions, and not the least of them is faulty nutrition. Furthermore, these tragedies often befall children whose parents are able to purchase the best food available.

Almost every food we eat has been tinkered with in one way or another. The majority of children today, especially those living in cities, have never once tasted truly high-quality and nutritious fruits, vegetables, milk, or bread. Our foods are grown on depleted soils and are covered with poison sprays which fall on the ground and are carried with soil moisture into the heart of the food itself; they are shipped unknown distances, stored or held at room temperature for unknown periods, perhaps soaked, canned, or frozen. Our meats, eggs, and milk, produced by animals receiving food far from ideal, lack the flavor and nutritive value they should have; the meat may be frozen and lose valuable juices on thawing; the milk may be pasteurized or canned. Our cereals are precooked, puffed, flaked, exploded, or otherwise tortured, their nutritive value largely being lost in the process. The number of refined and health-destroying foods on the market is appalling, and almost every radio or television program blares at your children to eat them. Many of the nutritive losses are small and unavoidable, but they are nevertheless real; the sum total of all losses is tremendous indeed. The cumulative effect of eating such food over a period of years can mean only one thing: a lower degree of health than is your child's birthright.

For these reasons nutritional supplements must now be used, whereas formerly they were not needed. They are your safeguards. Supplements, however, should never be used as an excuse for poor food. They are necessary today only because much of the best food available is of extremely poor quality. Also supplements must not be overemphasized. It is the ordinary food served day after day which largely determines health. No mother who becomes at all careless in planning menus or in selecting or preparing food can expect her children to be healthy.

Take the bull by the horns. One of the most encouraging trends today is the number of young parents who are buying a small plot of land, enriching the soil, and growing much of their own food. If it is possible for you to join their ranks, do so. There are many excellent books on the subject * which may help you. Raising your own food will assure your family of a higher degree of health. For example, vegetables grown in soil to which humus has been added have been found to contain as much as 400 per cent more minerals than the same variety of vegetable grown on nearby soil lacking humus.[3] The vitamin and protein content of foods is also increased when the biological life of the soil is improved.

If you cannot raise your own food, try to find where in your community you can obtain foods grown under good agricultural management. Such foods may not be available, but they never will be available until mothers demand them, or as long as

* Thomas J. Barrett, *Harnessing the Earthworm* (Sun Valley, California: Dr. T. J. Barrett, 1948).

Sir Albert Howard, *Soil and Health* (New York: Devin Adair Co., 1947).

Ehrenfried Pfeiffer, *Bio-Dynamic Farming and Gardening* (New York: Anthroposophic Press, 1943).

J. I. Rodale, *Pay Dirt* (New York: Devin Adair Co., 1949).

Leonard Wickenden, *Make Friends with Your Land* (New York: Devin Adair Co., 1949).

[3] Herbert C. White, "Progress Report of Foods for Life," *The Newsletter Journal, American Academy of Applied Nutrition,* 3 (1950), 4.

mothers are content to buy the poor-quality produce sold in most markets.

In case you do not enjoy baking bread at home, ask a baker to make the kind of bread you want. Several friends of mine have asked bakers to make bread of wheat germ and freshly stone-ground, whole-wheat flour free from harmful preservatives. The baker who supplies our community with such bread * sells several hundred loaves daily. Also he makes of the same ingredients the most delicious hamburger rolls I have ever tasted and excellent cookies containing blackstrap molasses, wheat germ, powdered milk, and unrefined flour. Dozens of similar products could be baked with health-building ingredients if mothers would only ask for them. It is a great satisfaction to know that every slice of bread your child eats is supplying him with nutrients he needs. Can you see that such bread becomes available in your community?

Gradually stop buying or bringing into your house most of the foods which cannot build health. With the money you thus save, buy raw certified milk rather than pasteurized. Since unwholesome foods are more often eaten between meals than at meal-times, plan midmeals and shop for them. If your kitchen equipment is such that nutritive losses cannot be prevented, gradually replace it with better equipment. In case you have not done so already, study scientific methods of preparing foods and make sure you are not destroying or throwing away nutrients unnecessarily.

Last but perhaps most important, take the bull by the horns at

---

* To make 20 loaves of bread, combine and blend the following ingredients: 8 pounds water, 5 ounces salt, 8 ounces each bakers' yeast, blackstrap molasses, and bakers' honey; 1 pound shortening; keep all ingredients cold, or at 78° F. Add and mix at low speed for 2 minutes 15 pounds of stone-ground, whole-wheat flour having a gluten content not less than 16 per cent. Add more flour if needed. Add and mix 1 minute longer: 8 ounces powdered skim milk (dry milk solids) and 1 pound wheat germ. Take from mixer and let rise at 78° F. for 30 minutes. Scale, form into loaves, let rise in steam box at 98° F. for 40 minutes. Bake at 385° F. for 30 minutes. If ingredients are too warm during first rising or if wheat germ is added with first ingredients, the protein-digesting enzymes in the wheat germ will digest the gluten, and the bread will be heavy.

every meal, remembering that meals should be times of laughter and gaiety, when foods should be especially appetizing and delicious, and when friendships between parents and their children can be cemented into lasting values. Remember that parents should never be impolite in trying to teach their children politeness or good food habits or table manners. First make sure that your food can be enjoyed; then see that everyone enjoys it. If these simple rules are followed, raising healthy children can be fun. Let's have healthy children!

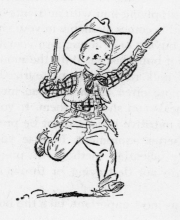

TABLE OF FOOD ANALYSIS

LIMITATIONS OF ANY TABLE OF FOOD ANALYSIS

Many physicians and nutritionists have criticized the use of tables of food analysis, some even arguing that such tables should not be published. The principal reason is that the nutrients in foods vary widely, depending upon numerous factors: the season in which the foods were grown; the amount of sunshine, rainfall, or water they received; the degree of ripeness or maturity when harvested; the method of fertilizing the soil; and particularly upon the amount of valuable bacteria, fungi, and humus in the soil and the minerals in the topsoil and subsoil. Thus potatoes or bunches of spinach grown in various localities have different nutritive values. Carrots, for example, have been analyzed which contain no vitamin A (carotene) whatsoever. The protein content of wheat, hence of breads and cereals, can vary from 3 to 22 per cent, depending upon the humus content of the soil. The nutritive value of milk, eggs, and meats vary with the diet of the animals which produced them. The losses which occur during harvesting, shipping, storing, processing, marketing, and preparing and cooking foods at home cause the nutritive values to vary much more. Although the analyses of foods in the following table were made at many universities and by reputable laboratories and are correct for the specific samples of food used, the foods you actually serve your family may have a far different analysis.

Another criticism is that such tables leave the impression that the nutrients listed are more important than those omitted: vitamins D, E, K, and P, the many B vitamins, and numerous minerals. One or more of these nutrients may be particularly vital to your individual health. Furthermore, even when a food is known to contain a certain nutrient, there is no assurance that it will be efficiently absorbed into your blood or not destroyed in the body or lost in the excreta.

The following table, however, may be used as a general guide in planning your menus provided you appreciate its limitations.

TABLE OF FOOD ANALYSIS ¶

In the following table, amounts of vitamin B_1 (thiamin), vitamin B_2 (riboflavin), vitamin C (ascorbic acid), calcium, phosphorus, and iron are given in milligrams (mg.). Vitamin A is in International, or United States Pharmacopeia, units.

With the exception of milk, average servings of food are given; weights and measures are of edible portions only. In case of cereals and legumes, raw weights are given with approximate cooked measure. Figures are for pasteurized milk and sulphur-dried fruits. Unless specified, vitamin and mineral contents are for uncooked foods, and allowances must be made for losses during cooking.

ABBREVIATIONS USED IN TABLE

* probably rich source   c. standard measuring cup   med. medium   sm. small
— amount insignificant   oz. ounce   ser. serving   st. stalk
.. no data available   in. inch   sl. slice   T. tablespoonful
av. average   lg. large   sq. square   t. teaspoonful

Food	Weight grams	Measure	Vitamins				Calcium mg.	Phosphorus mg.	Iron mg.	Protein grams	Calories
			A units	B_1 mg.	B_2 mg.	C mg.					
almonds	10	10 med.	0	.015	.010	1	25	45	0.3	2	65
apple	100	1 sm.	90	.036	.050	6	7	12	0.3	0	64
applesauce, sweetened	100	½ c.	60	.025	.075	5	10	18	0.4	0	150

Food											
apricots, dried	50	8 halves	6,850	.048	.250	0	16	30	0.8	1	102
apricots, fresh	100	6 halves	7,500	.033	.100	4	13	24	0.6	1	70
artichoke, Jerusalem	50	1 med.	200	.075	.015	10	20	47	0.4	1	32
asparagus, bleached	100	8 st.	0	.150	.065	12	21	40	1	2	20
asparagus, green	100	8 st.	1,100	.360	.065	20	21	40	1	2	20
avocado	100	½ med.	500	.120	.137	9	44	42	6.3	2	263
bacon, crisp	10	1½ sl.	0	.027	.007	0	0	3	0.1	2	53
banana	100	1 med.	300	.045	.087	10	8	28	0.6	1	85
barley, pearl	100	½ c. raw	0	.165	0	0	20	181	0.2	4	330
barley, whole	100	½ c. raw	—	2.200	:	0	51	400	4.7	4	310
beans, kidney, cooked	100	½ c.	300	.216	.210	0	46	152	0.6	6	88
beans, Lima, dry, cooked	90	½ c.	0	.300	.250	0	72	386	2.9	8	129
beans, Lima, green, cooked	100	½ c.	900	.225	.250	42	21	130	0.9	7	116
beans, navy, baked	100	½ c.	20	.150	.015	0	52	155	3.8	6	115
beans, string, green, cooked	100	¾ c.	950	.060	.100	8	55	50	1.1	2	43
beef broth	200	1 c.	0	:	:	0	0	:	:	4	30
beef, fat	113	4 oz. or 1 sl.	40	.135	.200	0	12	204	3	19	242
beef, lean	113	4 oz. or 1 sl.	60	.140	.262	0	13	214	3.4	22	190
beet greens, cooked	135	½ c.	22,000	.100	.500	50	94	40	3.2	2	28
beets	100	½ c.	50	.041	.037	8	28	42	2.8	2	40
blackberries	100	¾ c.	300	.025	.030	3	32	32	0.9	0	52

¶ Reprinted with permission from *Vitality Through Planned Nutrition* by Adelle Davis (rev. ed.; New York: The Macmillan Company, 1949).

Food	Weight grams	Measure	Vitamins				Calcium mg.	Phosphorus mg.	Iron mg.	Protein grams	Calories
			A units	B₁ mg.	B₂ mg.	C mg.					
blueberries	100	¾ c.	35	.045	.031	11	25	20	0.9	0	50
bologna	50	10 sl. sm.	0	.255	.200	0	40	102	4.2	8	109
brains, beef	113	4 oz.	54	.168	.360	18	16	340	5.3	11	127
bran, wheat flakes	25	1 c.	25	.240	.080	0	30	305	1.9	1	70
bread, rye	30	1 sl.	—	.066	..	0	12	74	0.6	3	76
bread, white, milk	30	1 sl.	10	.015	.020	0	14	32	0.2	3	72
bread, white, roll	50	1 lg.	12	.024	.025	0	12	40	0.2	4	100
bread, whole-wheat, 100%	30	1 sl.	10	.180	.100	0	22	102	1.1	3	75
broccoli, flower	100	¾ c.	6,000	.120	.350	65	64	105	1.3	2	35
broccoli, leaf	100	¾ c.	30,000	.120	.687	90	262	67	2.3	3	35
broccoli, stem	100	¾ c.	2,000	..	.187	..	83	35	1.1	2	35
Brussels sprouts	100	¾ c.	400	.180	.090	130	27	121	2.1	4	55
buckwheat, whole	100	5 T.	..	.660	..	0	24	306	2.6	12	240
butter ¶	10	2 t., 1 sq.	225	.012	0	0	1	1	0	0	77
buttermilk	960	1 qt.	400	.300	1.850	0	1,200	960	—	30	400
cabbage, inside leaves	100	1 c. raw	0	.078	.075	50	46	34	0.2	2	28
cabbage, Chinese	100	1 c. raw	5,000	.036	.462	50	400	72	2.5	2	30

cabbage, green	1 c. raw	100	160	.090	.150	50	429	72	2.8	2	28
cake, chocolate	1 sl.	50	160	.015	.030	0	21	48	0.4	3	200
cake, devil's food	1 sl.	50	150	.019	.037	0	11	101	2.9	3	177
cake, sponge	1 sl.	25	160	.036	.006	0	18	55	0.8	2	72
candy, chocolate	1 piece	15	—	0	0	0	0	0	0	—	45
candy, chocolate nut	1 bar	40	—	..	..	0	0	—	0	5	219
candy, gumdrop	1 lg.	10	0	0	0	0	0	0	0	1	36
candy, marshmallow	1 av.	6	0	0	0	0	0	0	0.	—	20
candy, milk chocolate	1 bar	50	—	0	0	0	10	—	0	4	282
candy, mint	1 piece	6	—	0	0	0	0	0	0	0	20
candy, peanut brittle	2 x 3 x ¼ in.	25	0	.045	.030	0	5	26	0.4	3	115
cantaloupe (see melon)											
carrots	½ c. diced	100	4,500	.070	.075	5	45	41	0.6	1	30
cashew nuts	20 nuts	30	0	*	.076	0	16	160	..	6	202
cauliflower	¾ c.	100	10	.085	.090	75	122	60	0.9	2	25
celery, bleached	4 st.	100	20	.030	.015	5	78	46	0.5	1	19
celery, green	4 st.	100	640	.030	.045	7	98	46	0.8	1	19
celery root	½ c.	100	..	..	..	2	47	71	0.8	3	38
cereal, whole-wheat, cooked	⅔ c.	100	7	.140	.030	0	10	98	1.4	3	100
chard, leaves, cooked	½ c.	100	15,000	.450	.165	37	150	50	3.1	2	25
cheese, American	2 x 1 x 1 in.	40	1,000	.018	.200	0	380	274	0.4	12	160
cheese, Cheddar	2 T.	30	500	.045	.650	0	254	181	0.1	7	100

¶ Summer butter may supply 5 to 10 units of vitamin D per square.

Food	Weight grams	Measure	Vitamins				Calcium mg.	Phosphorus mg.	Iron mg.	Protein grams	Calories
			A units	B₁ mg.	B₂ mg.	C mg.					
cheese, cottage	100	½ c.	180	.018	.250	0	240	263	—	20	100
cheese, cream	20	1 T.	3,500	.010	.112	0	127	104	—	2	75
cheese, Swiss	30	1 sl.	660	..	.150	0	330	281	0.4	10	135
cherries, stoned	100	12 lg.	259	.051	—	12	19	30	0.4	1	90
chestnuts, fresh	20	6 nuts	0	.048	..	0	7	19	0.8	—	37
chicken	113	4 oz.	0	.140	.180	0	14	232	3.1	18	125
chocolate malted milk	350	12 oz.	2,260	.333	.532	0	390	306	1.1	11	514
chocolate milk shake	350	13 oz.	1,240	.168	.432	0	390	300	0.9	10	472
chocolate pudding ¶	125	½ c.	592	.015	.150	0	149	164	—	5	272
chocolate, sweetened	30	1 oz.	0	.025	..	0	27	130	0.7	—	170
clams	113	6, or ¾ c.	20	.021	.015	15	95	93	4.2	14	100
Coca-cola	200	7 oz.	0	0	0	0	0	0	0	0	135
cocoa †	150	1 c.	300	.030	.150	0	186	62	0.4	5	135
coconut, dried	20	3 T.	..	.015	.025	0	12	31	0.4	1	130
cod-liver oil, U.S.P.‡	15	1 T.	10,000	0	0	0	0	0	0	0	100
cod fish	113	4 oz.	10	.150	.192	0	12	120	0.6	16	70
coffee, liquid	200	1 c.	0	0	0	0	0	0	0	0	0

Food	Grams	Measure									
collards, cooked	100	½ c	6,300	.130	*	70	207	75	8.4	3	41
cookie, molasses	25	1 lg.	—	—	..	0	39	25	1.5	2	100
corn, canned, yellow	100	½ c.	900	.130	.120	4	6	103	0.4	4	120
corn, on cob, yellow	100	1 med.	860	.209	.055	8	8	103	0.4	3	90
corn oil	11	1 T.	0	0	0	0	0	0	0	0	100
corned beef	113	4 oz.	..	..	*	0	13	119	6.8	16	196
cornflakes	20	¾ c.	0	.020	.020	0	10	38	0.1	2	100
cornmeal, white	100	½ c.	0	.110	.082	0	16	152	0.5	8	270
cornmeal, yellow	100	½ c.	500	.110	.100	0	16	152	0.9	8	272
cottonseed oil	11	1 T.	0	0	0	0	0	0	0	0	100
crab	113	⅔ c.	..	.135	.420	12	17	181	0.1	16	80
crackers, graham	20	2	0	.048	..	0	4	20	0.2	2	84
crackers, soda	12	2 lg.	0	0	0	0	2	10	0	1	53
cranberries, sauce	100	¾ c.	30	0	0	6	13	11	0.4	—	300
cream, table, 20%	60	4 T.	510	.030	.090	0	45	40	—	2	105
cream, whipping, 40%	60	4 T.	1,020	.030	.090	0	38	36		1	240
cream soup, spinach §	150	¾ c.	4,800	.087	.150	2	157	144	3.5	5	150
cream soup, tomato §	150	¾ c.	1,100	.096	.150	3	130	140	0.6	4	141
cucumbers ¶	100	1 med.	35	.060	.054	12	10	21	0.3	1	15

¶ 100 grams milk, ¼ egg.
† 100 grams milk.
‡ Supplies 1,700 units of vitamin D.
§ ½ c. milk, whole, 3 T. vegetable.

Food	Weight grams	Measure	Vitamins				Calcium mg.	Phosphorus mg.	Iron mg.	Protein grams	Calories
			A units	B₁ mg.	B₂ mg.	C mg.					
custard ¶	130	½ c.	918	.048	.225	0	134	175	0.7	7	126
dandelion greens, cooked	100	½ c.	20,000	.190	.270	100	84	35	6	3	45
dates, dried, stoned	100	15 med.	155	.060	.054	0	70	56	3.5	2	347
doughnuts	100	2	190	.018	.087	0	21	55	1.6	7	481
duck	113	4 oz.	..	.360	..	0	10	200	2.3	21	159
egg, whole	50	1 av.	600	.065	.150	0	32	112	1.5	6	75
egg white	30	1 white	0	.005	.050	0	4	5	0	3	12
egg yolk	20	1 yolk	600	.060	.100	0	28	107	1.5	3	58
eggplant	100	½ c.	70	.042	.036	10	11	31	0.5	1	15
endive	100	10 st.	15,000	.058	.072	20	104	39	1.2	1	8
escarol (chicory)	100	¾ c.	23,000	.075	.250	7	29	27	1.5	1	20
farina, raw, refined	20	2 T.	0	.010	0	0	5	25	0.1	2	72
figs, dried	30	2 sm.	15	.015	.032	0	54	38	0.7	1	103
figs, fresh	50	2 lg.	50	.037	.030	1	26	18	0.4	1	42
fish (average)	113	4 oz.	16	.148	.220	0	12	128	1.6	21	140
flour, buckwheat	113	1 c.	0	.300	..	0	11	193	1.3	6	387
flour, rye	113	1 c.	0	.171	.072	0	18	289	1.4	9	388

flour, soybean	1 c.	113	..	.650	.370	0	200	450	7.4	37	379
flour, wheat, fortified †	1 c.	113	0	.450	.220	0	270	90	3.3	10	354
flour, wheat, refined	1 c.	113	0	.070	.054	0	20	90	1	10	354
flour, wheat, whole-grain	1 c.	113	42	.450	.160	0	45	423	5	12	361
frankfurters	2 links	113	0	*	..	0	7	117	1.6	14	244
gelatin, dried	1 T.	10	0	0	0	0	0	17	..	8	84
gingerale	7 oz.	200	0	0	0	0	0	0	0	0	90
goose	4 oz.	113	..	.150	..	0	10	175	2.4	22	153
gooseberries	¾ c.	100	150	.150	..	25	40	50	0.4	1	37
grapefruit, fresh	½ med.	100	20	.070	.060	45	21	20	0.2	0	36
grapefruit juice, fresh	1 c., or 8 oz.	240	50	.075	.144	108	42	40	0.4	1	72
grapefruit juice, canned	1 c., or 8 oz.	240	50	.065	.144	72	42	40	0.4	1	100
grape juice, canned	½ c.	100	0	.020	.020	0	11	10	0.3	0	60
grapes	1 sm. bunch	100	25	.030	.024	3	19	35	0.7	1	80
guavas	1	100	200	.156	.105	125	15	16	3	1	56
haddock	4 oz.	113	7	.120	.198	0	18	197	0.5	17	72
halibut	4 oz.	113	0	.120	.222	0	20	200	1	19	121
ham	4 oz.	113	0	.800	.225	0	13	54	5.7	20	248
heart, beef	4 oz.	113	..	.660	.900	4	12	129	3.7	17	96
herring	4 oz.	113	200	.120	.330	0	23	246	0.6	19	394
hominy, white	½ c.	100	0	.054	0	0	12	112	0	0	355

¶ ½ c. milk, whole, ½ egg.
† Fortified flour means that iron, thiamin, and niacin have been added to refined flour.

| Food | Weight grams | Measure | Vitamins | | | | Calcium mg. | Phosphorus mg. | Iron mg. | Protein grams | Calories |
			A units	B₁ mg.	B₂ mg.	C mg.					
honey	25	1 T.	0	0	0	1	0	6	0.1	0	101
huckleberries	100	½ c.	100	.045	.021	8	25	20	0.2	1	60
ice cream, commercial	100	½ c.	170	.036	.150	0	202	74	0.6	2	208
jams	50	4 t.	0	0	—	0	—	—	—	0	176
jellies	50	4 t.	0	0	—	0	—	—	—	0	156
jello ¶	200	¾ c.	0	0	0	0	0	0	0	2	112
kale, cooked	100	½ c.	20,000	.189	.570	96	195	67	2.5	4	45
ketchup, tomato	20	1 T.	—	.	.	10	3	8	0.2	—	21
kidney, beef	113	4 oz.	1,100	.300	2.520	10	9	182	4.2	15	137
kohlrabi	100	½ c.	..	.030	.120	50	195	60	0.7	2	32
lamb chop	113	2 chops	0	.300	.330	0	21	180	3.3	20	359
lamb, roast	113	4 oz.	0	.225	.320	0	21	180	1.7	22	225
lamb's-quarters (greens)	100	½ c.	19,000	.180	.600	82	180	70	2.6	4	55
lard	30	2 T.	2	.051	.009	0	0	0	0	0	270
leeks	100	½ c.	20	.150	..	24	58	56	0.6	2	40
lemon juice	50	4 T.	0	.024	.002	25	11	6	0.3	0	20
lentils, cooked	100	½ c.	200	.378	.390	0	20	77	1.7	9	115

	Weight	Measure									
lettuce, green	100	10 leaves	2,000	.075	.150	7	49	28	1.5	1	10
lettuce, white	100	¼ head	125	.051	.062	5	17	40	0.5	1	10
lime juice	50	¼ c.	65	:	:	18	28	17	—	0	20
liver, beef	113	4 oz. or 1 sl.	9,000	.300	2.500	30	11	368	9.2	20	140
liver, calf	113	4 oz. or 1 sl.	7,000	.250	2.250	25	8	420	9.4	23	148
liver, chicken	113	4 oz. or ½ c.	8,000	.210	:	25	:	:	:	20	130
liver, lamb	113	4 oz. or 1 sl.	9,000	.300	2.500	20	8	400	7.9	20	120
liver, pork	113	4 oz. or 1 sl.	6,000	.450	2.500	12	10	370	8.1	20	150
lobster, canned	100	½ c.	:	.150	.156	5	18	188	0.9	16	84
loganberries, canned	100	1 c.	:	.033	:	35	35	24	1.3	1	64
macaroni, white, cooked	100	¾ c.	0	.005	0	0	24	119	0.1	3	130
macaroni, whole-wheat	100	¾ c.	0	.410	.160	0	45	423	5.1	4	130
malted milk, dry	30	2 T.	2,040	.330	.200	0	:	:	:	2	82
mandarin (orange)	100	2 sm.	150	.080	.150	46	45	21	0.5	0	61
margarine	28	1 oz.	:	0	0	0	—	3	0.1	—	261
marmalade, orange	25	1 T.	:	0	:	0	8	3	0.1	—	85
mayonnaise	15	1 T.	—	:	.007	0	2	—	—	—	100
melon, cantaloupe	150	½ sm.	900	.090	.100	50	32	30	0.5	1	44
melon, honey dew	150	¼ med.	100	:	:	90	:	:	:	0	35
melon, watermelon	300	1 med. ser.	450	.180	.084	22	33	9	0.6	0	90
milk, condensed	100	½ c.	680	.096	.420	0	300	235	0.3	9	326
milk, dried, skim	100	10 T., or ½ c. rounded	0	.340	1.960	0	1,220	850	0.5	35	350

¶ Made with water.

Food	Weight grams	Measure	Vitamins				Calcium mg.	Phosphorus mg.	Iron mg.	Protein grams	Calories
			A units	B₁ mg.	B₂ mg.	C mg.					
milk, evaporated	100	½ c.	680	.056	.390	0	250	200	0.5	8	150
milk, fresh, dry feed	960	1 qt.	800	.240	1.500	2	1,100	930	1.6	33	660
milk, fresh, green feed	960	1 qt.	3,500	.600	2.100	12	1,220	960	2.8	33	660
milk, fresh, skim	960	1 qt.	30	.300	1.925	11	1,220	960	0.4	34	370
milk, fresh, whole, average	960	1 qt.	2,920	.300	1.900	10	1,200	930	2.2	33	660
milk, goat	960	1 qt.	1,630	.547	.950	12	1,152	960	2	32	672
molasses, blackstrap	20	1 T.	0	.490	.580	0	259	35	9.6	1	52
molasses, blackstrap, fortified ¶	20	1 T.	0	1.049	.580	0	259	35	9.6	1	52
molasses, dark, unrefined	20	1 T.	0	0	0	0	40	8	1.4	—	57
molasses, light (corn syrup)	20	1 T.	0	0	0	0	2	1	0	0	59
muffin, bran	35	1 lg.	20	.150	.040	0	26	24	0.4	1	120
muffin, wheat-germ †	35	1 lg.	25	.450	.062	0	26	24	0.6	1	120
mushrooms	100	¾ c.	0	.160	.070	2	14	98	0.7	4	36
mustard greens, cooked	100	½ c.	11,000	.138	.450	125	291	84	9.1	2	25
mutton, leg	113	4 oz.	0	.360	.330	0	10	270	3	20	191
oatmeal, cooked	20	½ c.	0	.190	.075	0	4	79	1.4	4	80

okra	100	½ c.	440	.126	..	17	72	62	2.1	2	24
olives, green	25	5	50	0	0	0	40	4	0.6	—	35
olive oil	15	1 T.	0	0	0	0	0	0	0	0	135
onions, dry	100	2 sm.	0	.042	.125	2	41	47	0.3	1	45
onions, fresh	100	4 med.	60	.042	.125	7	41	47	0.4	1	42
orange	100	1 med.	190	.090	.075	50	44	18	0.4	—	50
orange juice, canned	240	1 c. or 8 oz.	460	.225	.230	80	90	45	0.9	1	110
orange, fresh	240	1 c. or 8 oz.	460	.200	.230	120	90	45	0.9	1	110
oysters	100	7 med.	250	.225	.540	3	33	156	5.8	6	50
parsley	50	½ c.	8,000	.057	..	70	23	15	9.6	20	24
parsnips	100	½ c.	100	.120	..	40	60	76	1.7	2	65
peaches, dried	25	3 halves	1,000	.020	.050	0	12	19	0.6	1	77
peaches, white, raw	100	3 halves	100	.025	.065	6	10	19	0.2	1	50
peaches, yellow, canned	100	2 lg. halves	600	.024	.060	8	10	19	0.3	1	50
peaches, yellow, raw	100	1 lg.	1,000	.025	.065	9	10	19	0.3	1	50
peanut butter	34	2 T.	120	.210	.200	0	24	192	0.6	9	203
peanuts	20	18 nuts	70	.225	.110	0	15	73	0.4	5	110
pears	100	1 med.	17	.030	.060	4	15	18	0.3	0	60
peas, dried, cooked	20	½ c.	520	.142	.162	0	17	80	2.8	12	173
peas, fresh, cooked	100	½ c.	1,500	.390	.250	20	28	127	2	7	100
pecans	33	10 lg.	90	.100	.075	0	29	112	0.8	3	229

¶ Fortified by adding 30 milligrams of thiamin to a pint of molasses.
† 1 T. per muffin.

Food	Weight grams	Measure	Vitamins A units	Vitamins B₁ mg.	Vitamins B₂ mg.	Vitamins C mg.	Calcium mg.	Phosphorus mg.	Iron mg.	Protein grams	Calories
peppers, green	100	1 med.	700	.025	.025	125	12	28	0.4	1	25
peppers, pimiento	100	2 med.	500	..	..	200	6	26	0.4	1	23
persimmon, Japanese	150	1 lg.	1,600	0	0	40	22	21	0.2	2	116
pickles, cucumber	30	4 sm.	0	0	0	0	3	2	0.4	0	26
pie, apple ¶	100	1 lg. sl.	45	.018	.025	2	8	39	0.2	3	274
pie, apricot ¶	100	1 lg. sl.	3,700	.018	.050	3	11	45	0.4	3	274
pineapple, canned	100	2 sl.	25	.075	.025	10	8	26	0.1	0	65
pineapple, fresh	100	⅔ c.	30	.100	.025	38	8	26	0.2	0	57
pineapple juice, canned	240	1 c. or 8 oz.	60	.105	.060	25	20	69	0.2	0	129
plums	100	3 med.	130	.120	.056	5	20	27	0.5	1	80
potatoes, sweet	100	1 med.	3,600	.155	.150	25	19	45	0.9	3	130
potatoes, white, baked	100	1 med.	0	.200	.075	20	13	53	1.5	3	92
potatoes, white, raw	100	1 med.	0	.220	.075	33	13	53	1.5	3	90
potatoes, yam	100	1 med.	5,000	.180	.360	6	44	50	1.1	2	150
pork chops	113	4 oz. or 2 chops	0	.540	.312	0	16	180	2.5	14	340
pork chops, lean, cooked	113	4 oz.	0	.800	.225	0	18	180	5.7	23	240
pork sausage	113	6 links	0	.445	.300	0	7	116	1.6	10	402

prunes, dried	50	6 med.	1,500	.075	.325	4	27	57	1.5	2	173
pumpkin	100	½ c.	2,500	.056	.057	8	23	50	0.9	1	27
rabbit	113	4 oz.	0	.033	.072	0	20	201	0.6	20	192
radishes	100	15 lg.	0	.030	.054	25	21	29	0.9	1	22
raisins, seeded	30	¼ c.	30	.024	.050	0	20	44	0.9	1	105
raspberries, fresh	100	½ c.	260	.021	..	30	41	38	0.8	1	45
red-palm oil †	15	1 T.	50,000	0	0	0	0	0	0	0	100
rhubarb	100	½ c.	650	.024	.024	12	48	18	0.5	1	20
rice, brown, cooked	30	¾ c.	20	.190	.075	0	22	112	1.6	4	117
rice, polished, cooked	30	¾ c.	0	0	0	0	3	33	0.2	2	117
rice, puffed	10	½ c.	0	—	0	0	1	9	0.1	1	35
rutabagas	100	¾ c.	25	.075	.120	26	74	56	0.7	1	36
salsify (oysterplant)	100	2 roots	0	..	..	7	60	53	1.2	3	78
sardines, canned	50	4	200	.090	.370	0	170	195	1	13	103
sauerkraut	100	¾ c.	20	.008	..	5	45	29	0.3	2	28
salmon, canned ‡	113	4 oz.	250	.160	.100	0	26	250	1.2	22	203
scallops	113	4 oz.	..	..	..	3	115	338	3.0	16	81
shredded wheat	30	1 biscuit	0	.450	.130	0	15	141	1.5	3	108
shrimp	30	6 med.	25	.090	.065	2	32	78	0.9	8	27
soybeans, dried, cooked	100	½ c.	10	.525	.300	0	104	300	4	20	108

¶ 1½ c. fruit in a slice.
† Imported from India and Africa for making soaps and candles.
‡ Supplies 400 units of vitamin D.

Food	Weight grams	Measure	Vitamins				Calcium mg.	Phosphorus mg.	Iron mg.	Protein grams	Calories
			A units	B_1 mg.	B_2 mg.	C mg.					
soybeans, dried, uncooked	100	½ c.	25	1.312	.750	0	260	750	10.1	51	270
spaghetti, white, cooked	100	¾ c.	0	.005	0	0	25	26	0.2	3	127
spaghetti, whole-wheat, cooked	100	¾ c.	0	.410	.160	0	45	423	5.1	4	127
spinach, cooked	100	½ c.	11,000	.090	.312	30	78	46	2.5	2	25
squash, Hubbard, cooked	100	½ c.	4,000	.050	.075	3	19	15	0.5	1	46
squash, summer, cooked	100	½ c.	1,000	.040	.050	3	18	15	0.3	1	15
steak, beef	113	4 oz.	40	.150	.250	0	12	222	3.4	21	156
strawberries, fresh	100	½ c.	100	.025	..	50	34	28	0.6	1	30
sugar, brown	12	1 T.	0	0	0	0	15	2	0.4	0	50
sugar, white, refined	12	1 T.	0	0	0	0	0	0	0	0	50
syrup, maple	25	1 T.	0	0	0	0	25	4	0.8	0	64
sweetbreads, beef	113	4 oz.	..	.330	.510	0	15	595	1.6	14	310
tangerine	100	2 med.	300	.120	.054	48	42	17	0.2	1	42
tapioca, cooked	30	½ c.	0	0	.040	0	7	30	0.5	—	118
tea, liquid	200	1 c.	0	0	0	0	0	0	0	0	0

Food	Weight	Measure									
tomatoes, canned	100	½ c.	1,000	.075	.050	20	10	29	0.5	1	25
tomatoes, fresh	100	1 med.	1,500	.110	.050	25	11	29	0.4		20
tomato juice, canned	240	8 oz.	3,700	.195	.125	48	21	38	1	2	48
tongue, beef	113	4 oz.	..	.285	.264	0	8	200	6	16	226
turnips, cooked	100	½ c.	0	.062	.062	22	56	47	0.5	1	33
turnips, raw	100	1 med.	0	.065	.062	30	56	47	0.6	1	33
turnip tops, cooked	100	½ c.	11,000	.060	.450	130	347	49	3.4	2	28
tuna, canned	30	¼ c.	20	.030	.240	0	10	99	0.5	9	64
turkey	113	4 oz.	0	.150	.240	0	30	420	4.5	24	153
veal chops	113	4 oz. or 2 chops	0	.227	.298	0	12	220	2.8	19	209
veal, cutlets	113	4 oz.	0	.160	.360	0	15	228	3	20	184
veal, leg, cooked	113	4 oz.	0	.120	.400	0	16	240	3	23	180
walnuts, black	30	¼ c.	40	.110	..	0	..	..	2	0	222
walnuts, English	30	¼ c.	30	.130	..	0	22	100	0.5	5	197
watercress	25	¾ c.	1,250	.030	.090	15	40	11	0.8	0	6
wheatena, cooked	20	½ c.	7	.290	.030	0	10	77	1.1	2	73
wheat germ	100	½ c.	400	2.600	.750	0	71	1,050	7.5	24	220
white fish	113	4 oz.	..	.120	..	0	25	263	0.4	22	150
yeast, brewers', dried	45	1 heaping T. or 90 tablets	0	4.056	2.175	0	49	945	7.9	20	80

INDEX

Abscesses, breast, 7, 73; nutrition for, 74

Absorption, of calcium, 118; of foods, decreased by cathartics, 43; effect of frustration on, 154; of minerals and vitamins, 114, 115; of phosphorus, 118

Acetone, 38, 206-207; detected on breath, 206; in nail polish, 206

Acetone acidosis, 38, 206-207; remedy for, 207; symptoms of, 206

Acid, see Amino, Adenylic, Lactic, etc.

Acidosis, see Acetone acidosis

ACTH, 120

Adenoids, 225

Adenylic acid, 165

Air bubbles, 126, 130

Air inlets, in nursing bottles, 128-129, 130

Air swallowing, 155; as cause of colic, 195; prevention of, 150-152; problem with infants, 126, 141, 150; with mothers, 41

Albumin, formation of, 51; function of, 51; in blood, 51; in urine, 48, 52, 53; seriousness of lack of, 51, 53, 54-55

Alcoholic beverages, 65

Allergies, 185
as a scapegoat, 201
caused by egg, 174
emotional nature of, 237, 240, 250
fat babies and, 113
incidence of, in bottle-fed babies, 73, 115; in breast-fed, 73
prevention of, 229-242
relation of frustration to, 154, 159
relation to malnutrition, 237
rules for diets for, 234-235, 241
susceptibility to, caused by drugs, 207

Allergies (Cont.)
treated with vitamin C, 231; with other nutrients, 232-233
when antigens are unknown, 236
when severe, 240-241
without fear of, 248

Alpha tocopherol, see Tocopherol and Vitamin E

American cheese, see Cheese

American Indians, skeletal development of, 220

American Medical Association, 92; on mineral oil, 160; on Bang's disease, 121

Amino acids, essential ones lacking in gelatin, 25; in vegetables, 25; harmed by heat, 120; need for, 24; obtained from protein, 24; see also Methionine and Tryptophane

Anaphylactic shock, 230, 233

Anemia, 26, 35, 185; as warning of toxemia, 50; cause of fatigue, 40; caused by deficiency of B vitamins, 50; production of, by protein deficiency, 50, 55

Ankles, swelling of, 84, 51-52; danger of, 55; importance of, as a warning, 55; relation to protein deficiency, 51; treatment for, 52

Antagonism, during meals, 246, 249, 250-252; to cups, 168; to spoons, 168

Antibiotics, 121; dietary changes after giving, 209; effect on vitamins, 208

Antibodies, in breast milk (mature), 72; in colostrum, 82; made of protein, 24, 205; possible effect on allergies, 73, 234; production of, 161, 205

Anticolic bottles, 129

Before Conception

- for superior infant + to avoid illness

Prevent nausea with protein + Britain
(wheat germ, liver, yeast) — pg 24 + 29)
before and after pregnancy

Prevent miscarriage with Vit E (wheat germ oil)
before

See physician before conception for: blood count
blood pressure

Use any food which cannot build health —
Problems keep you from being hungry

During Pregnancy

Diet — pg 35

powdered skim milk .14 lb. (261)

Calcium on empty stomach — needed
esp. last 3 months + lactation —

Iron + copper — esp. last 2 mo. —
on empty stomach — tablets
during last half

Iodized salt important (mentally
defective
child)

Vit A — (carrots give more when cooked
fish - liver oil. 25,000 unit daily
(buy for cheapest price) afterward

Vit B — wheat germ, liver + yeast
needed everyday 'cus not stored
lost in urine so only 1 T. bet. each meal
liver at least weekly

cont. B yeast (175) produces B in the intestine

Vit. C — glass of orange juice daily (v.
C capsules... 15 mg ...
tablets (100 mg.) before ...

Vit D — nec. for cal. + phos.
25,000 unit capsule Tuesdays after ...

Vit E — 30 mg. daily

Vit K — injection in labor + baby after birth
.10 purchase (34) 5 mg. tablets / 1 daily last ...
every hr. during labor

Nausea — B vit. 100 mg of B6 at begin
tablets of 10 mg when needed
to prevent — 5 mg. tablets of B1 + B6 daily when
first preg.
eat protein + natural sug. or starch before ...
cheese + w.w. crackers. 15-30 before arising
100 mg of C with each meal if a ...
lose meals? 5-10 tablets of 100 mg C before bed
eat every 2 hrs.

) Fatigue — protein + Vit B — caused by anemia
liver daily + E concentrate + yeast

Heartburn (pg 41)
Constipation + Hemorroids — B vit (liver w...
daily
b. molasses — laxative   yeast, wh...
yogurt each meal with 1 tsp. milk sugar

Neuritis (pg 43)
Toxemia — 1 tsp. lecithin in tom. juice each meal
gain in weight, swollen ankles, head...
pain in stomach, visual disturb...
Vit B + protein (48)

Anemia — vit B (choline) or folic acid + B12
iron + protein
to correct — liver daily for 2 or 3 wks